CANCER Diet

COOKBOOK

For women

Over 50

My ultimate Anticancer Recipes that helped me manage and beat cancer

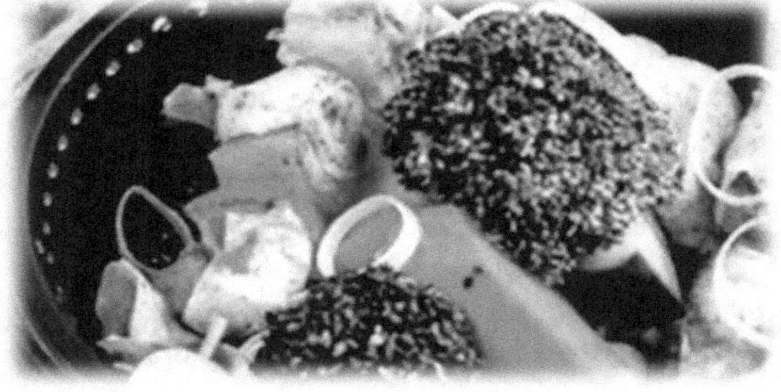

Dr. Grace Hester

A.kabod Publishing

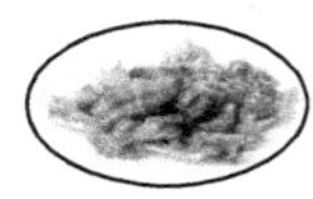 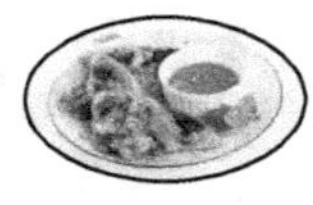 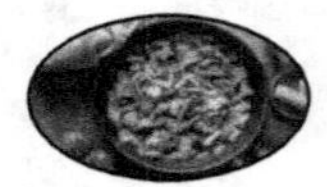

Copyright Page

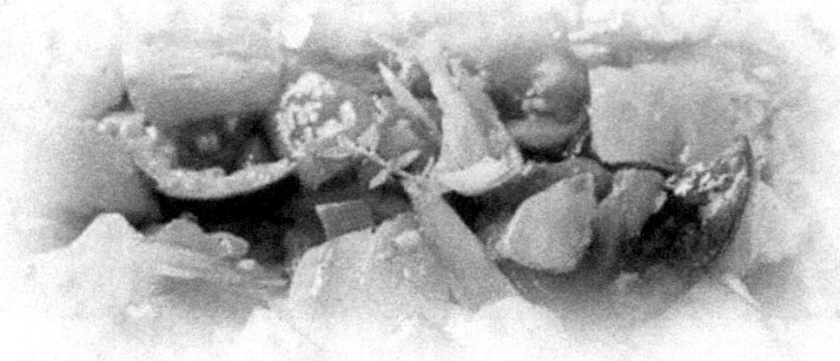

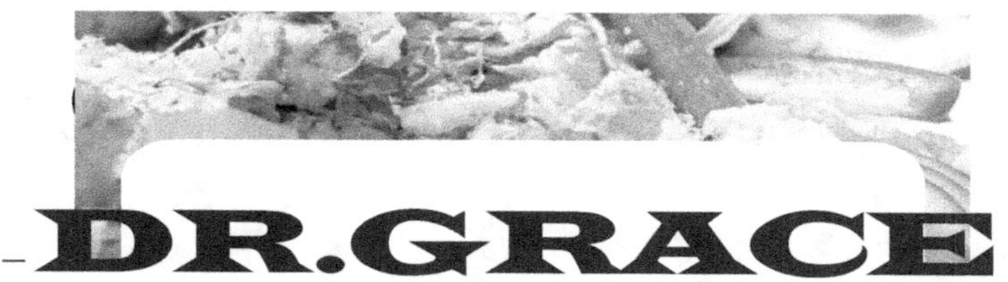

DR. GRACE HESTER

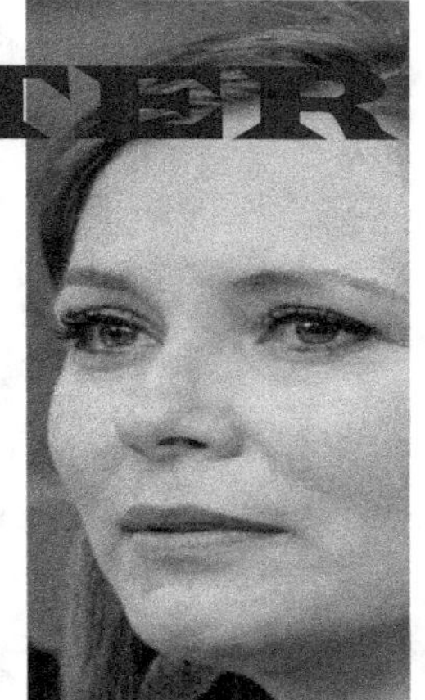

.Dr. Grace Hester stands at the intersection of health, passion, and culinary excellence. A distinguished medical professional and accomplished nutritionist, she seamlessly weaves together her expertise to create a holistic approach to well-being.

Dr. Hester earned her medical degree from the renowned Johns Hopkins School of Medicine, consistently ranked among the top medical schools globally. Her commitment to advancing healthcare led her to prestigious positions at the Mayo Clinic, where she honed her skills in internal medicine. Driven by a desire to explore the profound connection between nutrition and overall health, she furthered her education at the Culinary Institute of America.

— With a deep understanding of both medicine and nutrition, Dr. Hester embarked on a mission to inspire others to embrace a healthier lifestyle. Her culinary journey– led to the creation of a series of cookbooks that blend the art of cooking with the science of nutrition. Each recipe is a testament to her commitment to flavor, nourishment, and well-being.

B

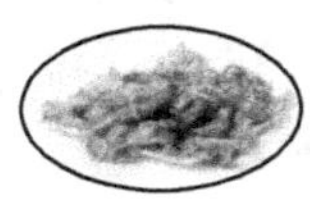
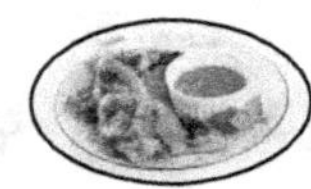
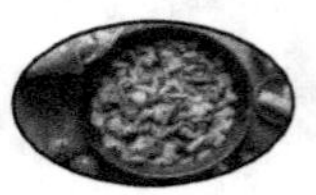

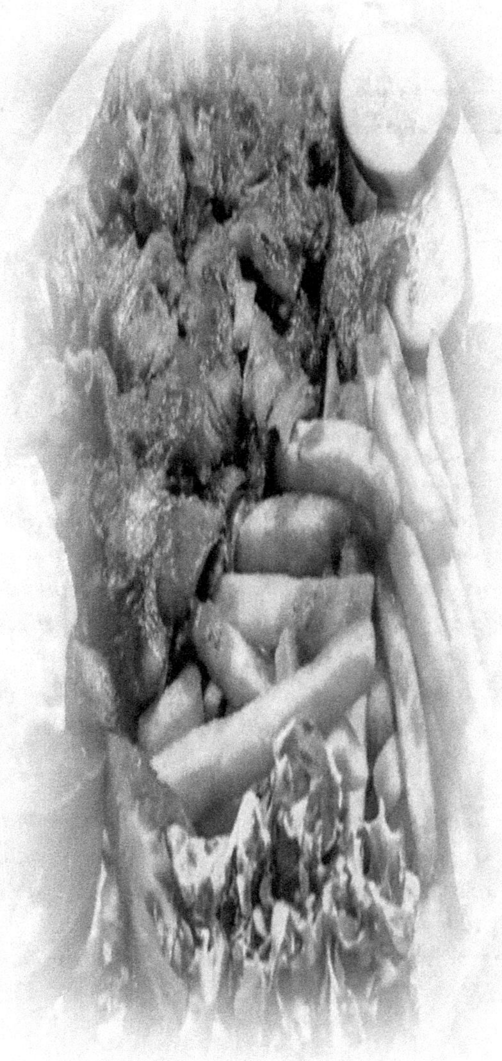

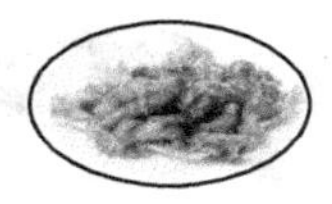 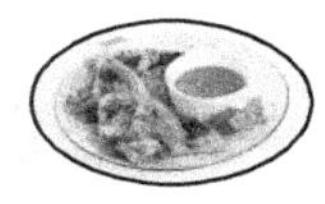 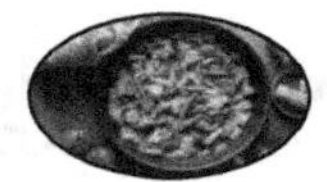

TABLE OF CONTENT

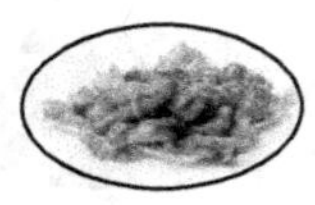 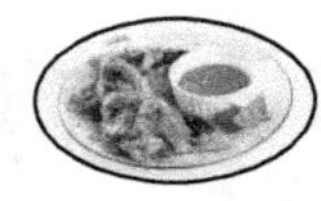 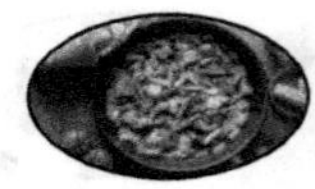

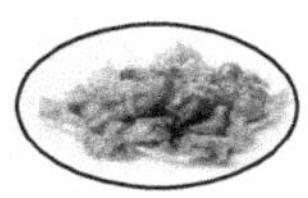 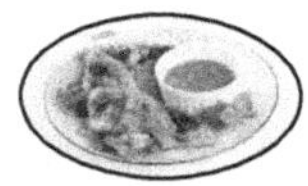 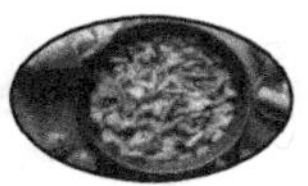

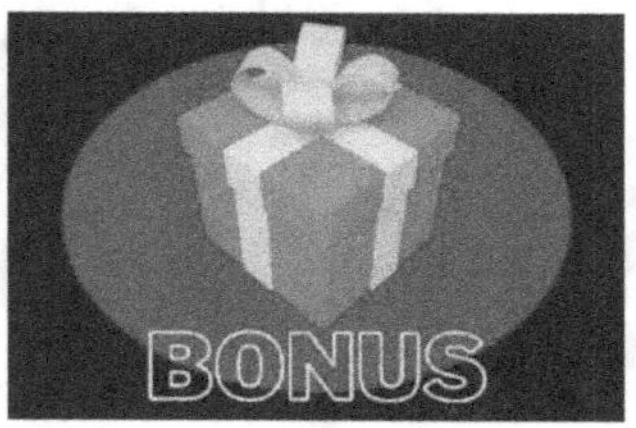

SCAN THE QR CODE TO GET YOUR FREE HOME
MADE GREEN SMOOTHIE RECIPE BOOK

Your 20 days meal planner is attached at the end of the
book. Enjoy!

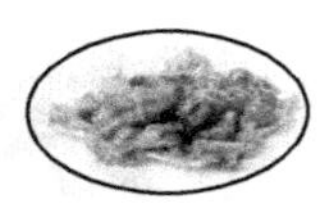 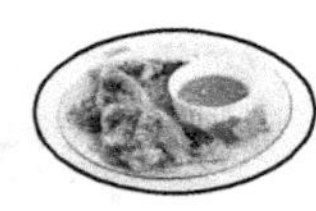 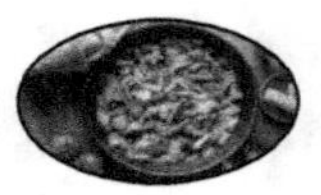

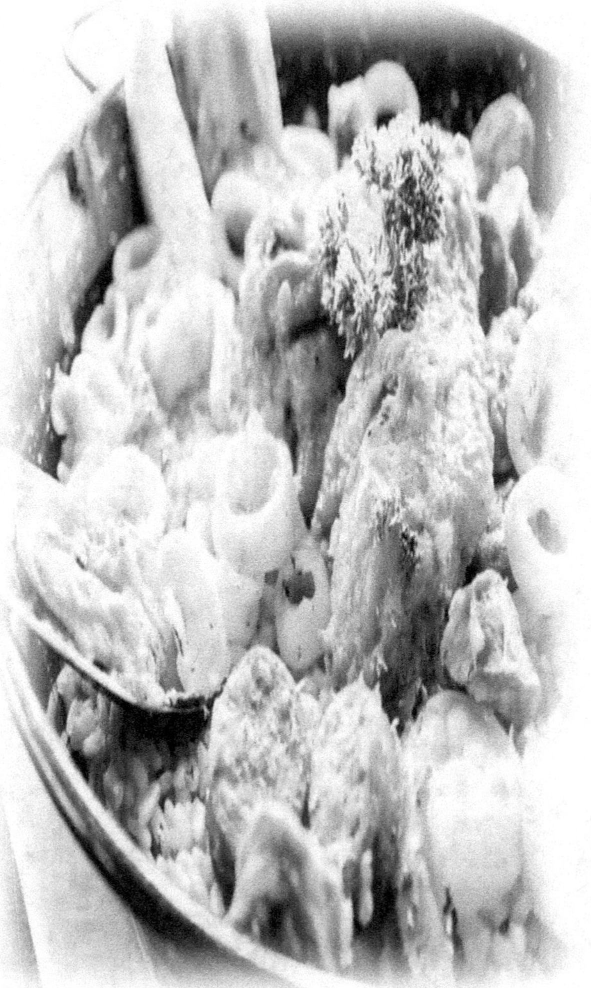

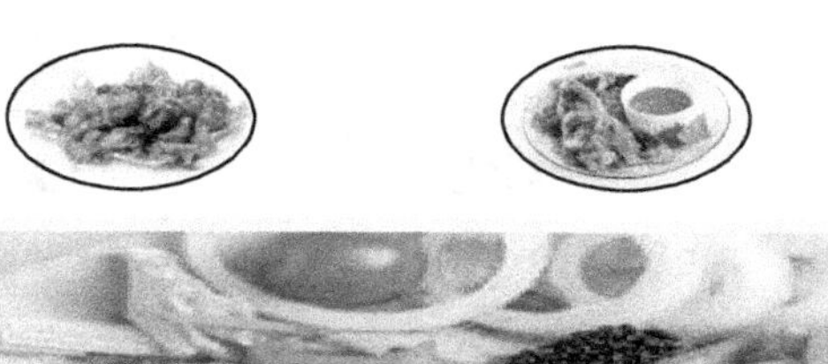

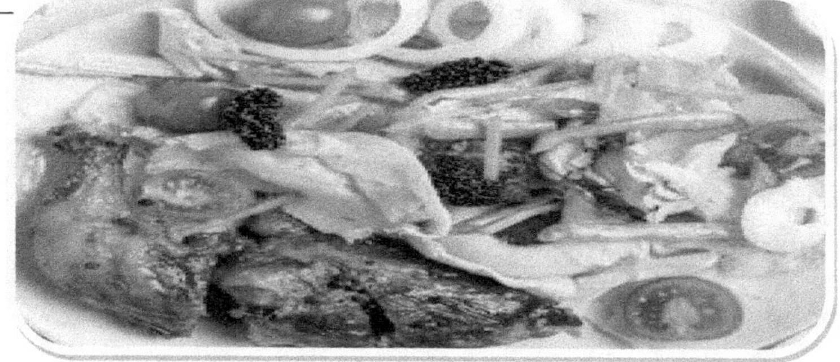

INTRODUCTION-

In the tapestry of life, we often encounter unexpected challenges that reshape our paths. For women over 50 facing the formidable adversary known as cancer, the journey becomes not only a battle against a formidable foe but a profound exploration of resilience, strength, and the healing power of nourishment.

This cookbook is more than a collection of recipes; it's a narrative woven with personal triumphs and a testament to the transformative nature of embracing an anticancer lifestyle. Within these pages, you'll find the culinary companions that fueled my own fight against cancer, recipes carefully curated to nourish not only the body but also the spirit.

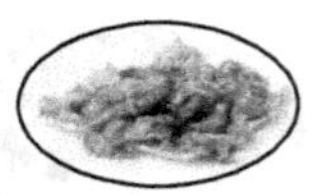 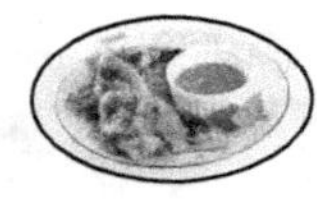 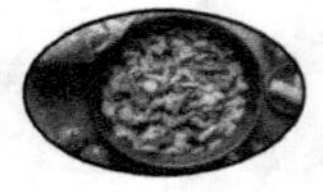

As I navigated the complexities of treatments and embraced the power of a cancer-conscious diet, I discovered that the kitchen could be a sanctuary, a place where healing ingredients and intentional cooking practices came together to support my well-being. From vibrant smoothies brimming with antioxidants to hearty meals infused with anti-inflammatory spices, each recipe tells a story of hope, strength, and the unwavering determination to overcome.

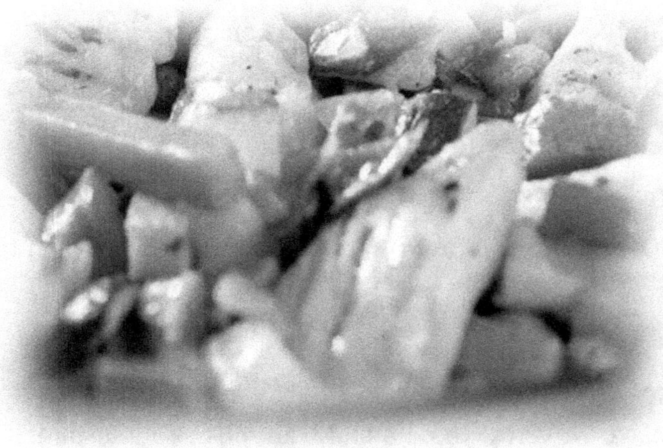

Whether you are on a personal journey or supporting a loved one, this cookbook invites you to embark on a culinary adventure designed to complement medical –

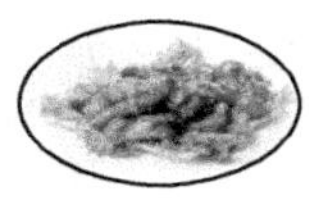 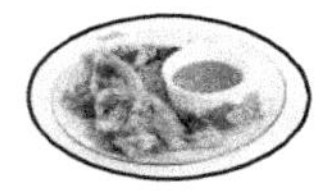 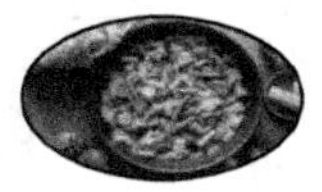

Interventions and foster holistic well-being. Each recipe is a small triumph, a step towards vitality, and a celebration of the joy that good food can bring—even in the face of adversity.

May this collection of anticancer recipes inspire and empower you on your own path to wellness. Together, let us savor the flavors of resilience and relish in the nourishment that fuels not only our bodies but our spirits on this remarkable journey.

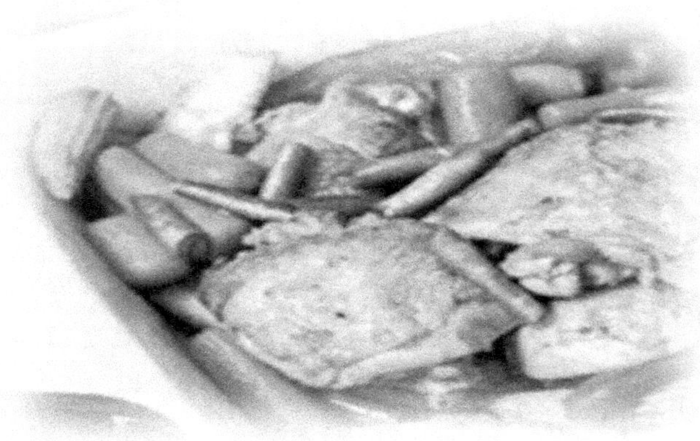

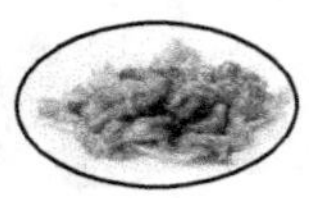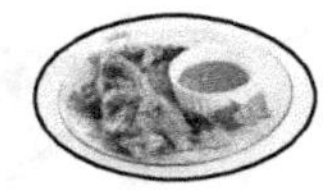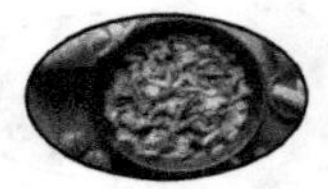

Recipe 1: Green Goddess Smoothie

INGREDIENTS:

- 1 cup kale, stemmed and chopped

- 1/2 cup spinach, fresh

- 1/2 cucumber, peeled and sliced

- 1/2 avocado, peeled and pitted

- 1 green apple, cored and chopped

- 1 cup coconut water

- 1 tablespoon chia seeds

- Ice cubes (optional)

INSTRUCTIONS:

1. Combine kale, spinach, cucumber, avocado, green apple, and coconut water in a blender.–

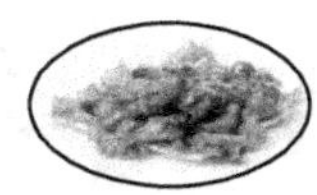 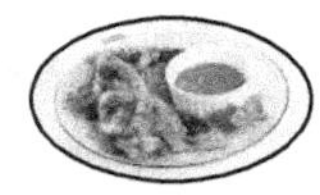 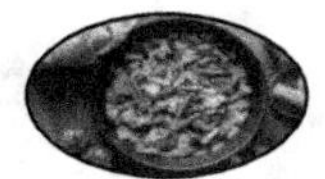

2. Blend until smooth.

3. Add chia seeds and blend again.

4. Pour into a glass over ice if desired.

5. Enjoy this nutrient-packed, cancer-fighting smoothie!

Recipe 2: Turmeric Quinoa Bowl

Ingredients:

- 1 cup quinoa, rinsed

- 2 cups vegetable broth

- 1 tablespoon coconut oil

- 1 teaspoon turmeric powder

- 1/2 teaspoon black pepper

- 1 cup broccoli florets–

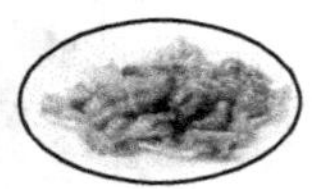 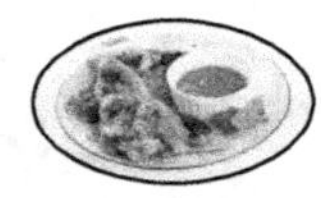 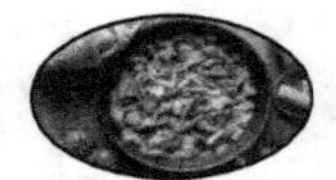

- 1 cup cherry tomatoes, halved

- 1/4 cup pumpkin seeds

- Fresh cilantro for garnish

Instructions:

1. . Gently mix the vegetable broth and quinoa in a good-sized saucepan. When quinoa is cooked, bring to a boil, then lower the heat and simmer

2. In a separate pan, heat coconut oil, turmeric, and black pepper.

3. Add broccoli and cherry tomatoes, sauté until tender.

4. Mix quinoa with the vegetable sauté.

5. Top with pumpkin seeds and garnish with fresh cilantro.

6. Serve warm and enjoy the anti-inflammatory benefits of turmeric.–

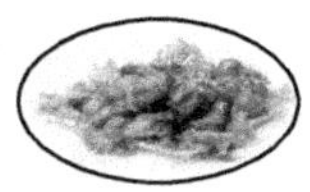 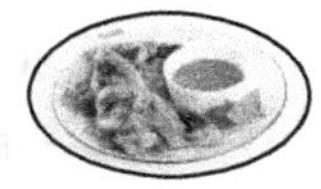 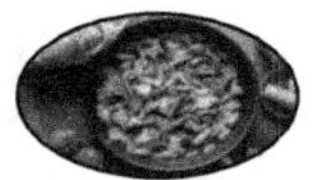

Recipe 3: Berry Avocado Salad

Ingredients:

- 2 cups mixed berries (strawberries, blueberries, raspberries)

- 1 avocado, sliced

- 2 cups mixed greens (kale, spinach, arugula)

- 1/4 cup walnuts, chopped

- 1 tablespoon flaxseed, ground

- Balsamic vinaigrette dressing

Instructions:

1. Toss mixed berries, avocado, and greens in a large bowl.

2. Sprinkle chopped walnuts and ground flaxseed over the salad.

3. Drizzle with balsamic vinaigrette dressing.

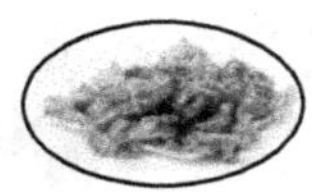 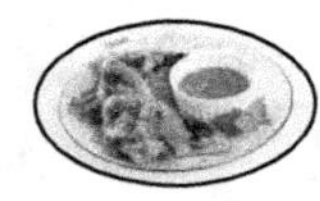 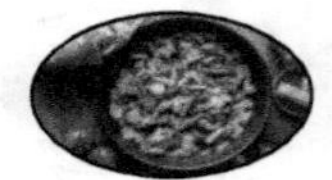

4. Gently toss until well combined.

5. Enjoy this refreshing and antioxidant-rich salad.

Recipe 4: Salmon and Broccoli Bake

Ingredients:

- 4 salmon fillets

- 2 cups broccoli florets

- 2 tablespoons olive oil

- 1 lemon, sliced

- 2 cloves garlic, minced

- 1 teaspoon dried dill

- Salt and pepper to taste

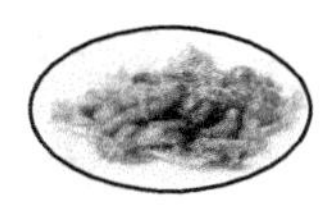 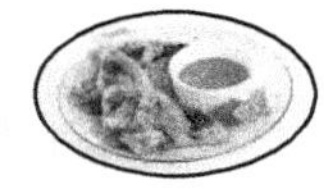 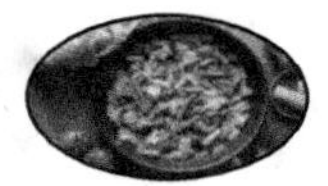

Instructions:

1. Preheat the oven to 400°F (200°C).

2. Place salmon fillets and broccoli in a baking dish.

3. Drizzle with olive oil and sprinkle minced garlic, dried dill, salt, and pepper.

4. Top with lemon slices.–

5. Continue baking for seventeen to twenty one minutes or until salmon changes color slightly.

6. Serve with a side of whole grains for a complete meal.

Recipe 5: Mushroom and Lentil Soup

Ingredients:

- 1 cup brown lentils, rinsed–

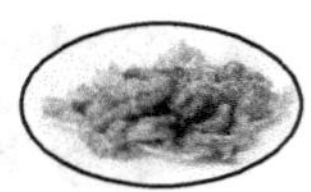 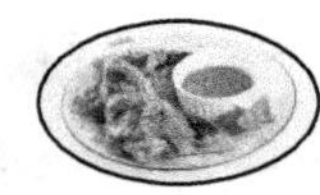 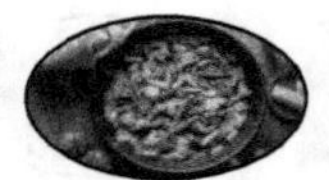

- 8 cups vegetable broth

- 1 tablespoon olive oil

- 1 onion, diced

- 2 carrots, sliced

- 2 celery stalks, chopped

- 8 oz mushrooms, sliced

- 2 cloves garlic, minced

- 1 teaspoon thyme

- Salt and pepper to taste

- Fresh parsley for garnish

Instructions:

1. In a large pot, heat olive oil and sauté onion, carrots, and celery until softened.

2. Add mushrooms and garlic, sauté for an additional 3-4 minutes.–

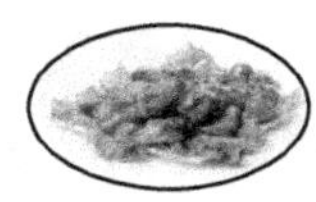 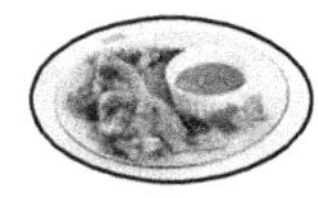 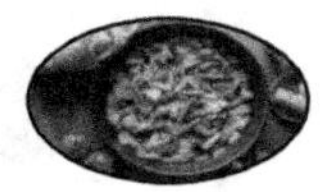

3. Pour in vegetable broth and add lentils.

4. Season with thyme, salt, and pepper.

5. Simmer until lentils are tender.

6. Garnish with fresh parsley before serving.

Recipe 6: Sweet Potato and Kale Stir-Fry

Ingredients:

- 2 sweet potatoes, peeled and cubed

- 2 cups kale, chopped

- 1 red bell pepper, sliced

- 2 tablespoons soy sauce

- 1 tablespoon sesame oil

- 1 tablespoon maple syrup–

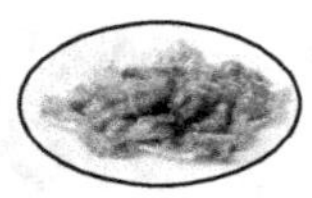 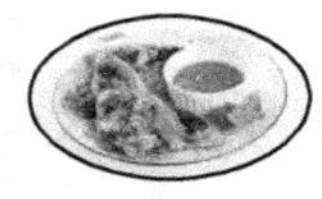 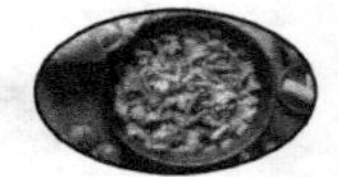

- 1 teaspoon ginger, grated

- 2 cloves garlic, minced

Instructions:

1. Steam sweet potatoes until just tender.

2. In a large pan, heat sesame oil and sauté garlic and ginger.

3. Add kale and red bell pepper, stir-fry until vegetables are crisp-tender.

4. Stir in sweet potatoes, soy sauce, and maple syrup.

5. Cook for an additional 2-3 minutes.

6. Serve over brown rice or quinoa.–

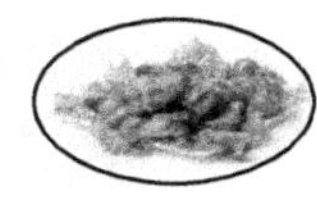 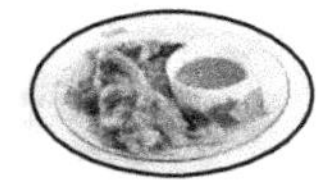 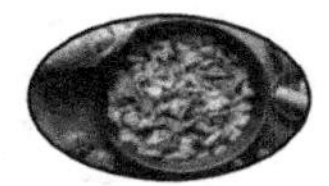

Recipe 7: Cauliflower and Chickpea Curry

Ingredients:

- 1 cauliflower, cut into florets

- 1 can chickpeas, drained and rinsed

- 1 onion, finely chopped

- 2 tomatoes, diced

- 1 can coconut milk

- 2 tablespoons curry powder

- 1 teaspoon turmeric

- 1 teaspoon cumin

- Salt and pepper to taste

- Fresh cilantro for garnish

—

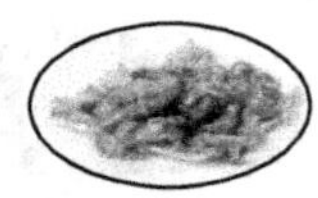 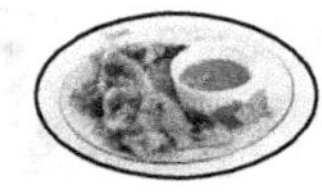 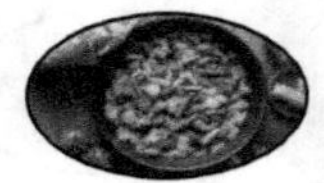

Instructions:

1. In a pot, sauté onion until translucent.

2. Add cauliflower, chickpeas, tomatoes, coconut milk, and spices.

3. Simmer until cauliflower is tender.

4. Season with salt and pepper.

5. Garnish with fresh cilantro before serving.

6. Enjoy this flavorful and hearty curry.

Recipe 8: Almond Butter and Banana Smoothie

Ingredients:

- 2 ripe bananas

- 2 tablespoons almond butter

- 1 cup almond milk–

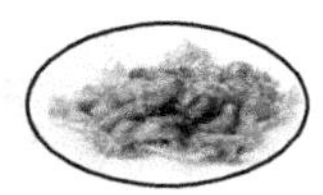 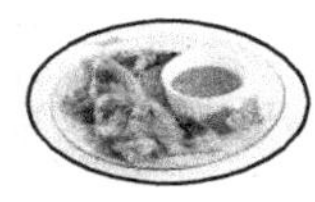 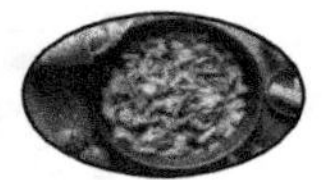

- 1/2 teaspoon cinnamon

- 1 tablespoon chia seeds

- Ice cubes (optional)

Instructions:

1. Place bananas, almond butter, almond milk, and cinnamon in a blender.

2. Blend until smooth.

3. Add chia seeds and blend again.

4. Pour into a glass over ice if desired.

5. A delicious and energy-boosting smoothie is ready to enjoy!–

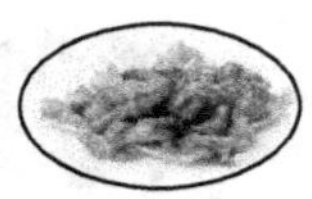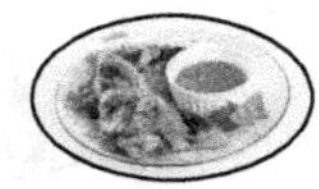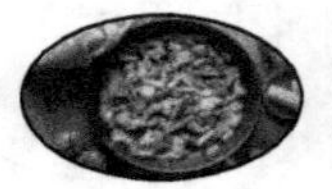

Recipe 9: Quinoa and Black Bean Stuffed Peppers

Ingredients:

- 4 bell peppers, halved

- 1 cup quinoa, cooked

- 1 can black beans, drained and rinsed

- 1 cup corn kernels

- 1 cup salsa

- 1 teaspoon cumin

- 1/2 teaspoon chili powder

- 1 cup shredded vegan cheese (optional)

Instructions:

1. Preheat the oven to 375°F (190°C).–

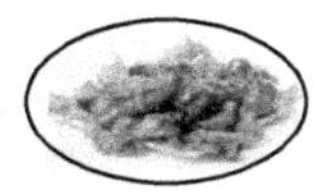 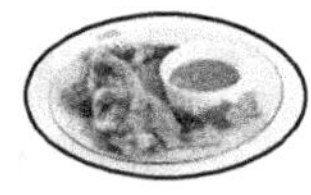 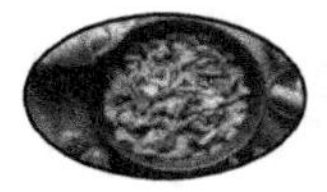

2. In a bowl, mix cooked quinoa, black beans, corn, salsa, cumin, and chili powder.

3. Stuff each bell pepper half with the quinoa mixture.

4. Top with vegan cheese if desired.

5. Bake for 20-25 minutes or until peppers are tender.

6. Serve with a side of guacamole.

Recipe 10: Blueberry Oatmeal Breakfast Bowl

Ingredients:

- 1 cup rolled oats

- 2 cups almond milk

- 1 cup blueberries

- 1 tablespoon honey

- 1/4 cup sliced almonds–

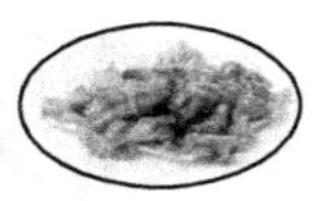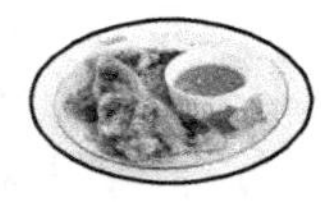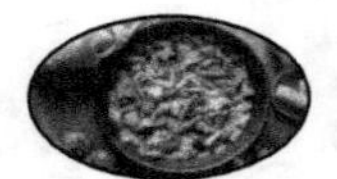

- 1/2 teaspoon vanilla extract

Instructions:

1. In a saucepan, combine rolled oats and almond milk.

2. Cook over medium heat until oats are creamy.

3. Stir in honey and vanilla extract.

4. Top with blueberries and sliced almonds.

5. Enjoy a nutritious and satisfying breakfast bowl to kick start your day!

Recipe 11: Spinach and Walnut Pesto Pasta

Ingredients:

- 8 oz whole-grain pasta

- 2 cups fresh spinach–

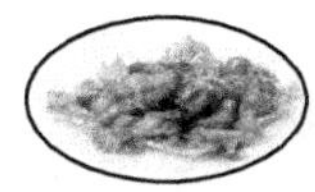 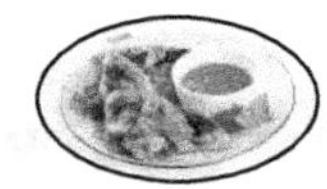 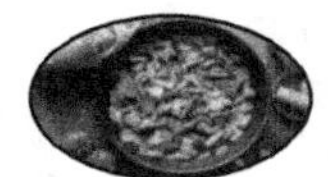

- 1/2 cup walnuts

- 1/2 cup nutritional yeast

- 2 cloves garlic

- 1/2 cup olive oil

- Salt and pepper to taste

Instructions:

1. Cook pasta according to package instructions.

2. In a food processor, blend spinach, walnuts, nutritional yeast, and garlic.

3. Gradually add olive oil until a smooth pesto is formed.

4. Toss the pesto with cooked pasta.

5. Season with salt and pepper.

6. Serve warm and savor the flavors of this nutrient-rich dish.–

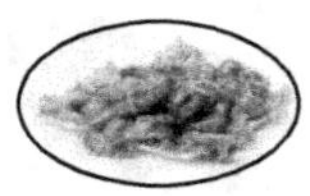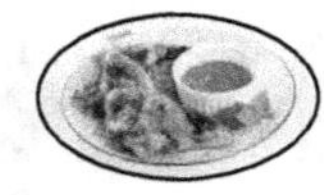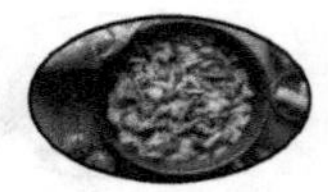

Recipe 12: Chia Seed Berry Parfait

Ingredients:

- Mixed berries, just a cup (such as blueberries, raspberries etc.)

- 1 cup coconut or almond yogurt

- 2 tablespoons chia seeds

- 1 tablespoon honey or maple syrup

- Granola for topping (optional)

Instructions:

1. In a bowl, mix chia seeds with yogurt and let it sit for 10 minutes.

2. Layer the chia-yogurt mixture with mixed berries in serving glasses.

3. Drizzle honey or maple syrup over each layer.

4. Repeat the layers until the glass is filled.

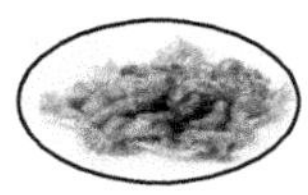 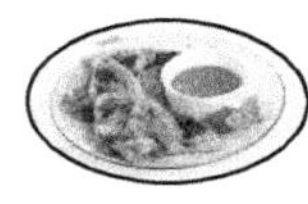 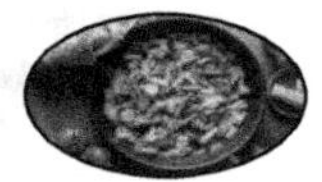

5. Top with granola if desired.

6. A delicious and healthy parfait is ready to be enjoyed!

Recipe 13: Roasted Brussels Sprouts with Balsamic Glaze

Ingredients:

- 1 lb trimmed Brussels sprouts.

- 2 tablespoons olive oil

- Salt and pepper to taste

- 2 tablespoons balsamic glaze

Instructions:

1. Preheat the oven to 400°F (200°C).

2. Brussels sprouts should be toss completely salt and pepper and with olive oil.

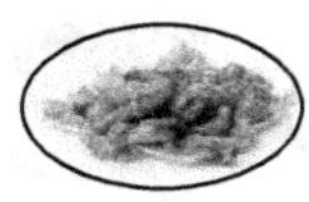 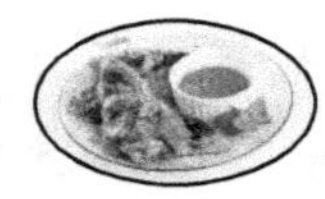 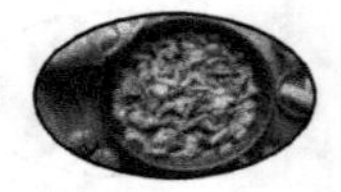

3. Roast in the oven for 20-25 minutes or until crispy.

4. Drizzle with balsamic glaze before serving.

5. A flavorful and nutritious side dish is ready to complement your meal.

Recipe 14: Lemon Garlic Grilled Chicken

Ingredients:

- 4 boneless, skinless chicken breasts

- 2 lemons, juiced and zested

- 3 cloves garlic, minced

- 2 tablespoons olive oil

- 1 teaspoon dried oregano

- Salt and pepper to taste

- Fresh parsley for garnish–

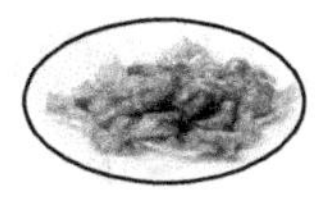 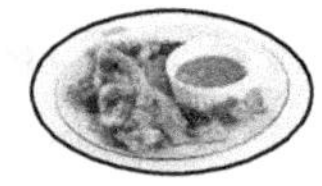 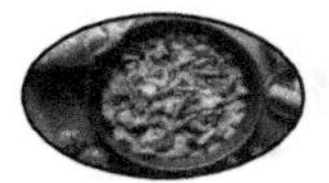

Instructions:

1. In a bowl, mix lemon juice, lemon zest, garlic, olive oil, oregano, salt, and pepper.

2. Marinate chicken breasts in the mixture for at least 30 minutes.

3. Grill chicken until fully cooked, about 6-8 minutes per side.

4. Garnish with fresh parsley before serving.

5. Enjoy a zesty and protein-packed main course.

Recipe 15: Cucumber and Dill Salad

Ingredients:

- 2 cucumbers, thinly sliced

- 1/4 cup red onion, thinly sliced–

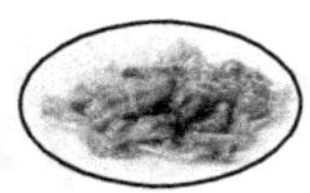 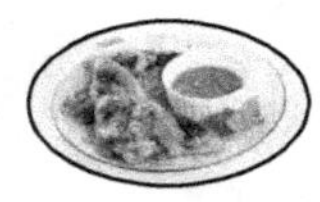 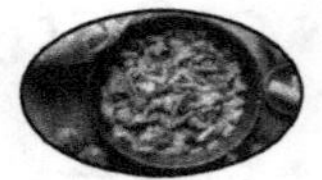

- 1/4 cup fresh dill, chopped

- 2 tablespoons apple cider vinegar

- 1 tablespoon olive oil

- Salt and pepper to taste

Instructions:

1. In a bowl, combine cucumbers, red onion, and dill.

2. Whisk together apple cider vinegar, olive oil, salt, and pepper.

3. Drizzle the cucumber mixture with the dressing and combine well.

4. Let it cool in the fridge for a minimum of half an hour prior to serving.

5. A refreshing and crisp salad awaits you.–

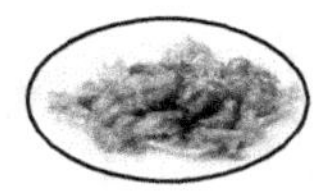 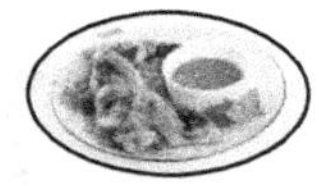 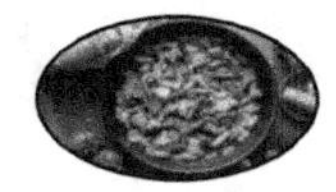

Recipe 16: Pumpkin and Lentil Soup

Ingredients:

- 1 can pumpkin puree

- 1 cup dry red lentils, rinsed

- 1 onion, diced

- 2 carrots, chopped

- 4 cups vegetable broth

- 1 teaspoon cumin

- 1/2 teaspoon nutmeg

- Salt and pepper to taste

- Pumpkin seeds for garnish

—

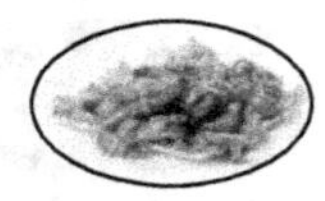 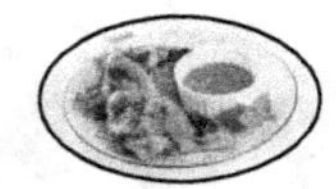 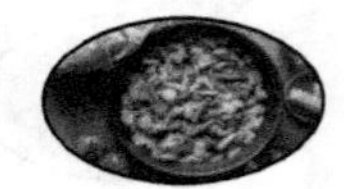

Instructions:

1. In a pot, sauté onion until translucent.

2. Add carrots, lentils, pumpkin puree, vegetable broth, cumin, and nutmeg.

3. Bring to a boil, then simmer until lentils are tender.

4. Season with salt and pepper.

5. Garnish with pumpkin seeds before serving.

6. Enjoy a warming bowl of this autumn-inspired soup.

Recipe 17: Quinoa and Veggie Stir-Fry

Ingredients:

- 1 cup quinoa, cooked

- 1 cup broccoli florets–

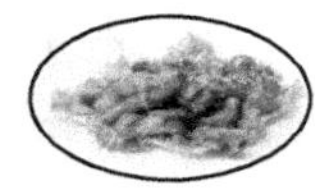 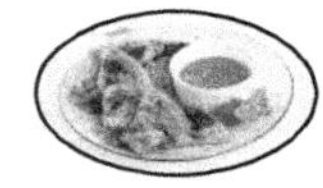 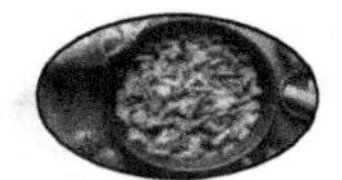

- 1 bell pepper, sliced

- 1 carrot, julienned

- 1 zucchini, sliced

- 2 tablespoons soy sauce

- 1 tablespoon sesame oil

- 1 teaspoon ginger, grated

- 2 cloves garlic, minced

Instructions:

1. Kindly heat sesame oil and ensure you sauté garlic and ginger in a large pan of your choice

2. Add broccoli, bell pepper, carrot, and zucchini.

3. Stir-fry until vegetables are crisp-tender.

4. Add cooked quinoa and soy sauce.

5. Toss until well combined.

6. Serve hot for a quick and nutritious meal.–

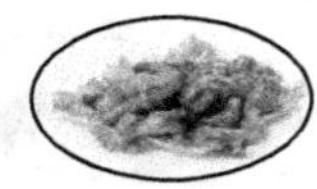 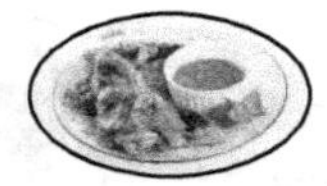 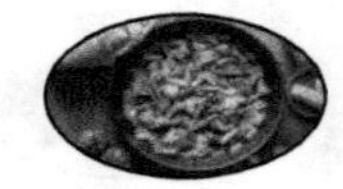

Recipe 18: Mango Avocado Salsa

Ingredients:

- 1 ripe mango, diced

- 1 avocado, diced

- 1/4 cup red onion, finely chopped

- 1/4 cup fresh cilantro, chopped

- Juice of 1 lime

- Salt and pepper to taste

- Jalapeño (optional, for heat)

Instructions:

1. In a bowl, combine mango, avocado, red onion, and cilantro.

2. Squeeze lime juice over the mixture.

3. Season with salt and pepper.

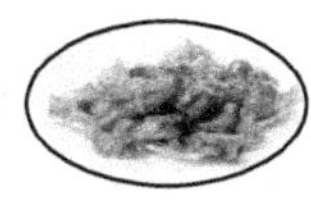 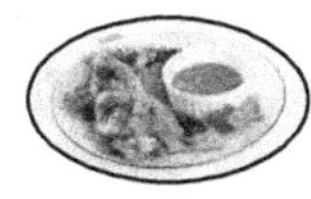 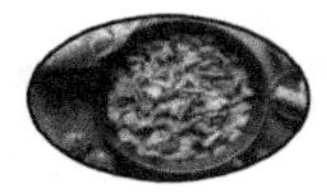

4. Add diced jalapeño if you like it spicy.

5. Mix well and let it sit for 10 minutes before serving.

6. A flavorful salsa that pairs perfectly with grilled proteins or as a snack.

Recipe 19: Tofu and Vegetable Skewers

Ingredients:

- 1 block firm tofu, cubed

- 1 zucchini, sliced

- 1 bell pepper, cut into chunks

- 1 red onion, cut into wedges

- 2 tablespoons soy sauce

- 1 tablespoon maple syrup

- 1 teaspoon garlic powder–

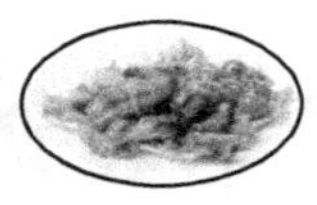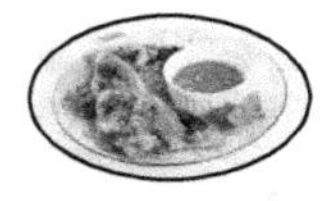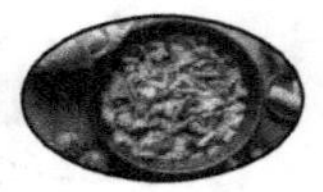

- 1/2 teaspoon smoked paprika

Instructions:

1. Preheat the grill or grill pan.

2. Thread tofu, zucchini, bell pepper, and red onion onto skewers.

3. In a bowl, mix soy sauce, maple syrup, garlic powder, and smoked paprika.

4. Brush the skewers with the sauce.

5. Grill for 10-12 minutes, turning occasionally.

6. Serve these flavorful skewers with your favorite side.–

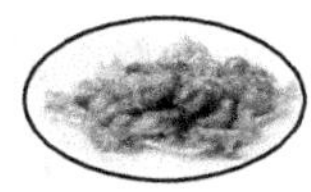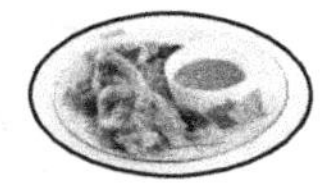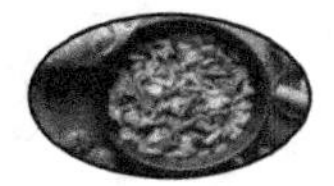

Recipe 20: Chocolate Avocado Mousse

Ingredients:

- 2 ripe avocados

- 1/2 cup cocoa powder

- 1/4 cup maple syrup

- 1 teaspoon vanilla extract

- Pinch of salt

- Fresh berries for topping

Instructions:

1. In a blender, combine avocados, cocoa powder, maple syrup, vanilla extract, and salt.

2. Blend until smooth and creamy.–

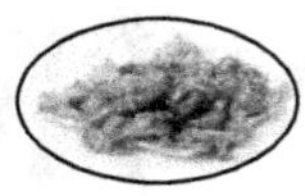 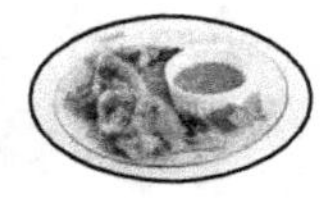 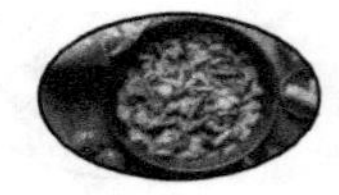

3. Chill the mousse in the refrigerator for at least 2 hours.

4. Spoon into bowls and top with fresh berries.

5. Indulge in this rich and guilt-free chocolate treat.

Recipe 21: Broccoli and Almond Stir-Fry

Ingredients:

- 2 cups broccoli florets

- 1/2 cup sliced almonds

- 1 red bell pepper, thinly sliced

- 2 tablespoons tamari or soy sauce

- 1 tablespoon rice vinegar

- 1 tablespoon sesame oil

- 1 teaspoon agave nectar–

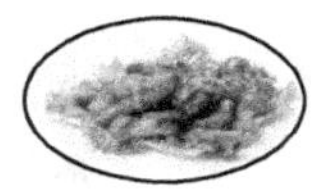 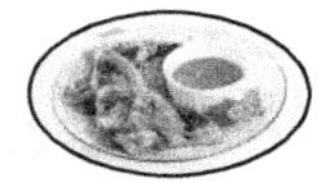 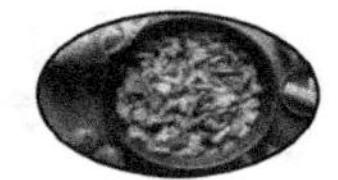

- 1 teaspoon cornstarch

- 2 cloves garlic, minced

- 1 teaspoon ginger, grated

Instructions:

1. In a bowl, whisk together tamari, rice vinegar, sesame oil, agave nectar, and cornstarch.

2. In a wok or large pan, heat the mixture and sauté garlic and ginger.

3. Add broccoli, sliced almonds, and red bell pepper.

4. Stir-fry until the broccoli is tender-crisp.

5. Pour the sauce over the stir-fry and toss until well coated.

6. Serve over brown rice or quinoa.–

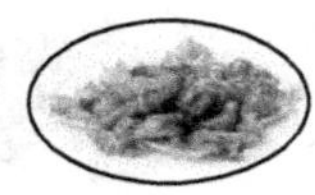 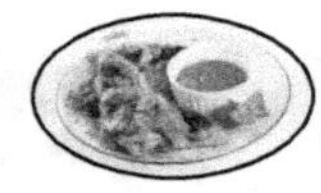 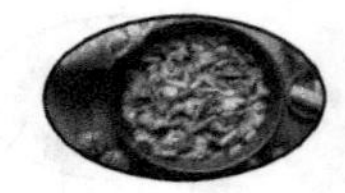

Recipe 22: Cabbage and Apple Slaw

Ingredients:

- 4 cups shredded green cabbage

- 2 apples, julienned

- 1/2 cup raisins

- 1/4 cup Greek yogurt

- 2 tablespoons apple cider vinegar

- 1 tablespoon honey

- 1 teaspoon Dijon mustard

- Salt and pepper to taste

—

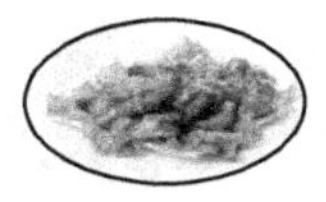 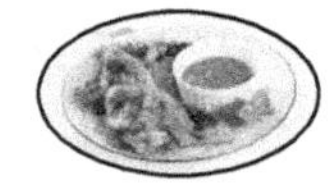 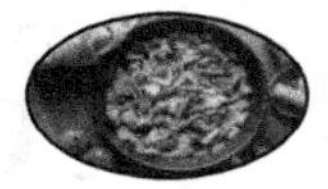

Instructions:

1. In a large bowl, combine shredded cabbage, julienned apples, and raisins.

2. Combine Greek yogurt, honey, Dijon mustard, apple cider vinegar, salt, and pepper in a another bowl

3. Pour the dressing over the cabbage mixture and toss until evenly coated.

4. Let it settle in the fridge for a minimum of half an hour before serving.

5. A refreshing and crunchy slaw that pairs well with grilled proteins.–

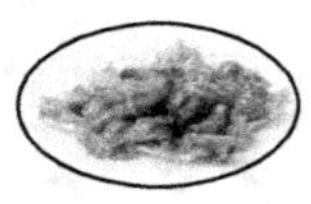 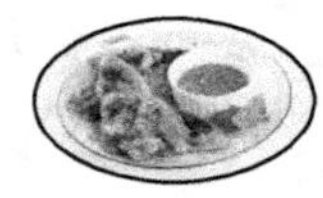 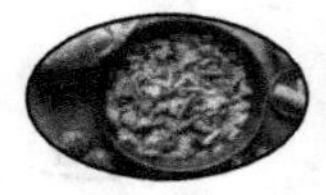

Recipe 23: Sesame Ginger Baked Tofu

Ingredients:

- One block of pressed and cubed extra-firm tofu

- 3 tablespoons soy sauce

- 1 tablespoon sesame oil

- 1 tablespoon rice vinegar

- 1 tablespoon maple syrup

- 1 teaspoon grated ginger

- 1 clove garlic, minced

- 1 tablespoon sesame seeds

- Green onions for garnish

—

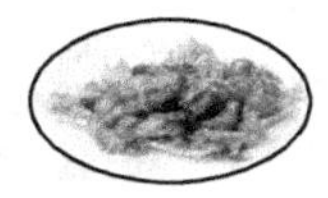 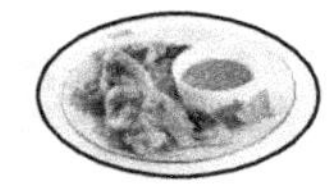 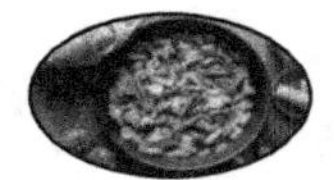

Instructions:

1. Preheat the oven to 400°F (200°C).

2. In a bowl, whisk together soy sauce, sesame oil, rice vinegar, maple syrup, grated ginger, and minced garlic.

3. Toss the tofu cubes in the marinade until well coated.

4. Place tofu on a baking sheet and sprinkle with sesame seeds.

5. .Bake for 25 to 30 minutes, rotating the cake after 15 minutes.

6. Before serving, garnish with finely chopped green onions.

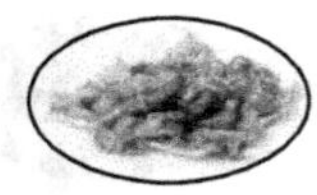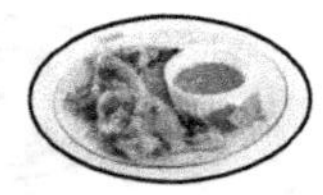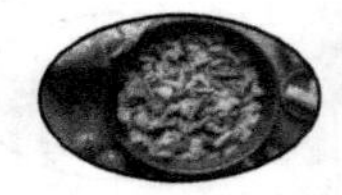

Recipe 24: Spaghetti Squash Primavera

Ingredients:

- One medium spaghetti squash, cut in half, and seeded

- 2 cups cherry tomatoes, halved

- 1 zucchini, sliced

- 1 yellow bell pepper, sliced

- 2 tablespoons olive oil

- 2 cloves garlic, minced

- 1 teaspoon dried oregano

- Salt and pepper to taste

- Fresh basil for garnish

—

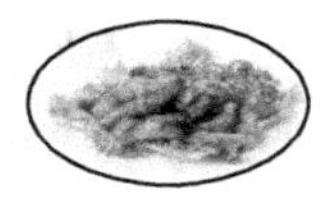 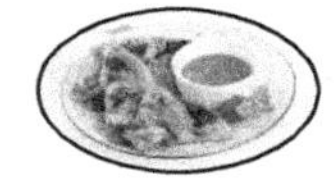 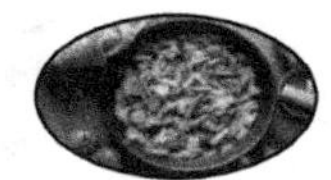

Instructions:

1. Preheat the oven to 400°F (200°C).

2. Drizzle olive oil over the cut side of the spaghetti squash and season with salt and pepper.

3. Place squash, cut side down, on a baking sheet and roast for 30-40 minutes until fork-tender.

4. In a pan, sauté garlic, cherry tomatoes, zucchini, and bell pepper until tender.

5. Scrape the spaghetti squash with a fork to create "noodles" and mix with the sautéed vegetables.

6. Garnish with dried oregano and fresh basil before serving.–

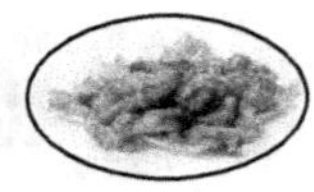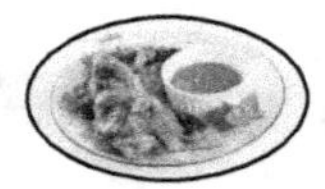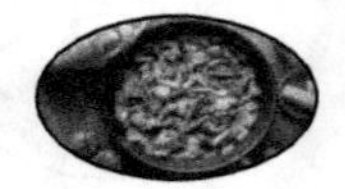

Recipe 25: Coconut Chia Seed Pudding

Ingredients:

- 1/4 cup chia seeds

- 1 cup coconut milk

- 1 tablespoon maple syrup

- 1/2 teaspoon vanilla extract

- Fresh fruit for topping (berries, kiwi, mango)

Instructions:

1. In a jar, combine chia seeds, coconut milk, maple syrup, and vanilla extract.

2. Stir well, cover, and refrigerate overnight.

3. In the morning of the day, please stir thoroughly.

4. Layer with fresh fruit in serving glasses.

5. Enjoy a creamy and nutritious chia seed pudding.

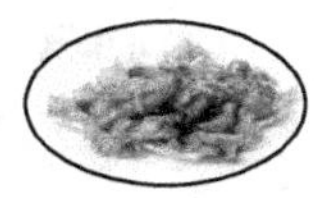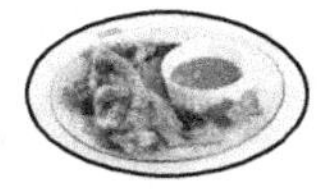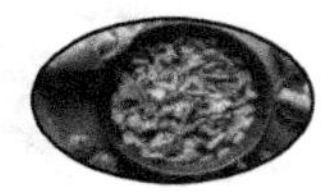

Recipe 26: Miso Glazed Eggplant

Ingredients:

- 2 large Japanese eggplants, sliced

- 2 tablespoons white miso paste

- 1 tablespoon rice vinegar

- 1 tablespoon sesame oil

- 1 tablespoon maple syrup

- 1 teaspoon grated ginger

- 1 clove garlic, minced

- Sesame seeds for garnish

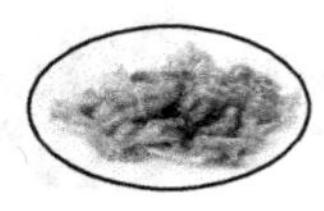 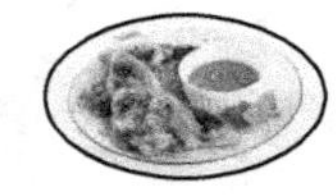 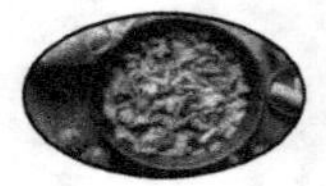

Instructions:

1. Preheat the oven to 400°F (200°C).

2. In a bowl, whisk together miso paste, rice vinegar, sesame oil, maple syrup, grated ginger, and minced garlic.

3. Brush the eggplant slices with the miso glaze and place on a baking sheet.

4. Bake for 20-25 minutes or until golden and tender.

5. Sprinkle with sesame seeds before serving.

6. Enjoy this flavorful and healthy side dish.–

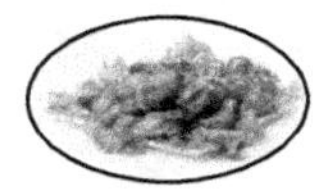 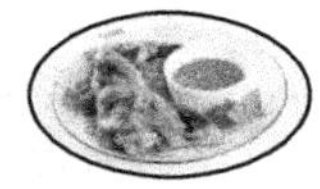 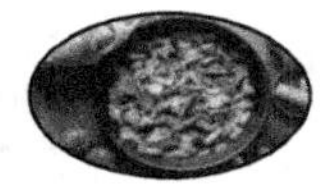

Recipe 27: Pomegranate and Walnut Quinoa Salad

Ingredients:

- 1 cup quinoa, cooked

- 1/2 cup pomegranate arils

- 1/2 cup chopped walnuts

- 1/4 cup fresh parsley, chopped

- 1/4 cup red onion, finely diced

- 2 tablespoons olive oil

- Juice of 1 lemon

- Salt and pepper to taste

Instructions:

1. In a bowl, combine cooked quinoa, pomegranate arils, walnuts, parsley, and red onion.

2. Drizzle with olive oil and lemon juice.

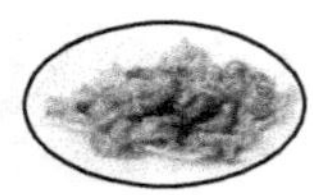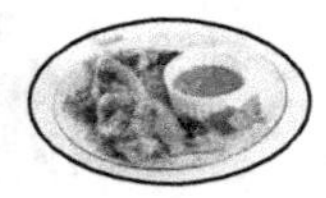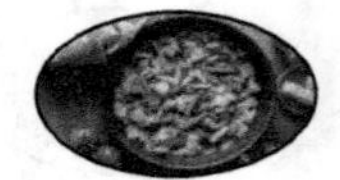

3. Season with salt and pepper.

4. Toss until well combined.

5. A vibrant and nutrient-packed salad is ready to be enjoyed.

Recipe 28: Stuffed Portobello Mushrooms

Ingredients:

- 4 large Portobello mushrooms, stems removed

- 1 cup quinoa, cooked

- 1 cup spinach, sautéed

- 1/2 cup cherry tomatoes, diced

- 1/4 cup feta cheese, crumbled

- 2 tablespoons balsamic glaze

- Fresh basil for garnish–

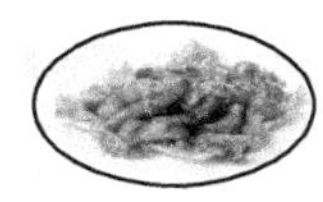 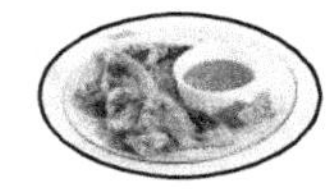 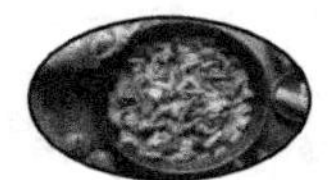

Instructions:

1. Preheat the oven to 375°F (190°C).

2. Place Portobello mushrooms on a baking sheet.

3. In a bowl, mix cooked quinoa, sautéed spinach, cherry tomatoes, and feta cheese.

4. Stuff each mushroom with the quinoa mixture.

5. Bake for 20-25 minutes until mushrooms are tender.

6. Drizzle with balsamic glaze and garnish with fresh basil.

Recipe 29: Carrot Ginger Immunity Soup

Ingredients:

- 4 cups carrots, chopped

- 1 onion, chopped–

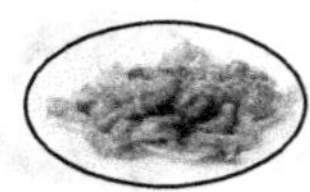 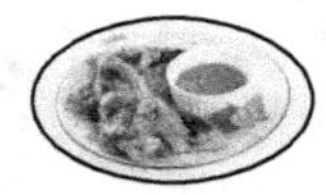 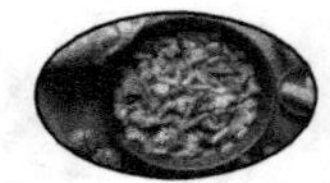

- 2 tablespoons fresh ginger, grated

- 4 cups vegetable broth

- 1 can coconut milk

- 1 tablespoon coconut oil

- 1 teaspoon turmeric

- Salt and pepper to taste

- Fresh cilantro for garnish

Instructions:

1. In a pot, sauté onion and ginger in coconut oil until softened.

2. Add chopped carrots, turmeric, vegetable broth, and coconut milk.

3. Bring to a boil, then reduce heat and simmer until carrots are tender.

4. Blend the soup until smooth.–

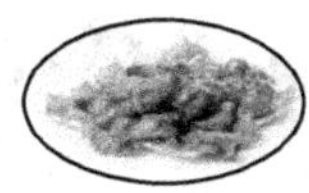 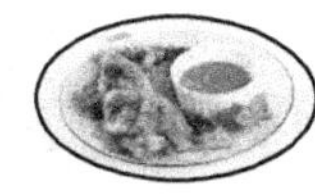 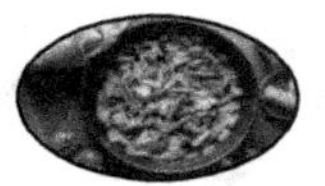

5. Season with salt and pepper.

6. Garnish with fresh cilantro before serving.

7. A comforting and immune-boosting soup to support your well-being.

Recipe 30: Avocado Chocolate Protein Smoothie

Ingredients:

- 1 ripe avocado

- 1 scoop chocolate protein powder

- 1 tablespoon almond butter

- 1 cup almond milk

- 1 tablespoon cacao powder

- 1 tablespoon maple syrup

- Ice cubes (optional)

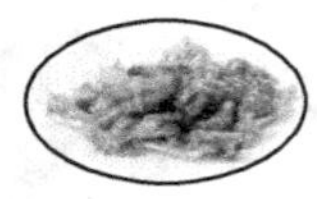 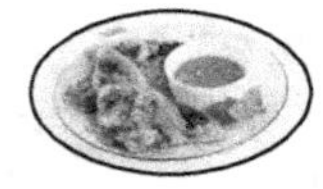 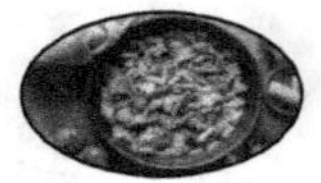

Instructions:

1. In a blender, combine avocado, chocolate protein powder, almond butter, almond milk, cacao powder, and maple syrup.

2. Blend until smooth.

3. Add ice cubes and blend again for a refreshing texture.

4. Pour into a glass and enjoy this nutrient-packed chocolate smoothie.

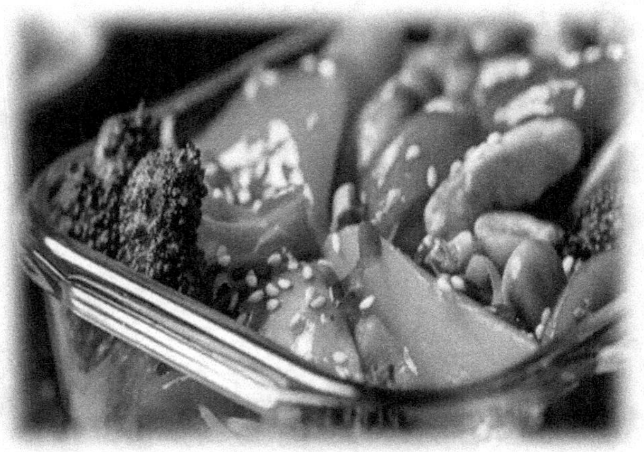

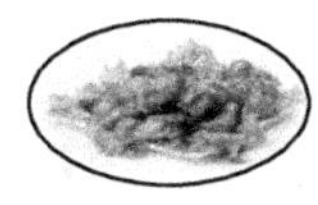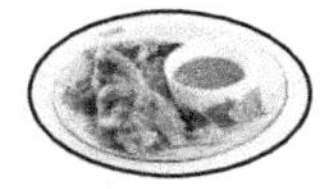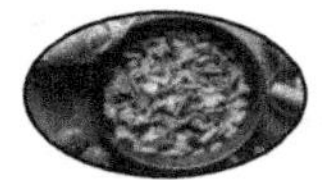

CONCLUSION

Embracing a Nourished Future

As we reach the final chapter of this anticancer cookbook for women over 50, I want to express my heartfelt gratitude for joining me on this transformative culinary journey. Each recipe shared within these pages represents more than a mere collection of ingredients; they are the embodiment of strength, hope, and the unwavering spirit that accompanies us through life's most challenging chapters.

In the world of cancer, victory is not solely measured in medical charts but in the daily choices we make to nourish our bodies and souls. The power of a well-balanced diet, rich in nature's healing elements, has been a guiding force in my own battle against cancer, and it is my sincere wish that it becomes a beacon of hope for you or your loved ones.

As you continue to explore and implement these anticancer recipes into your daily life, remember that this journey is a tapestry of small victories and daily choices. Cherish the

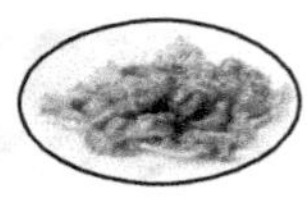 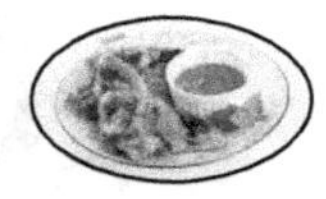 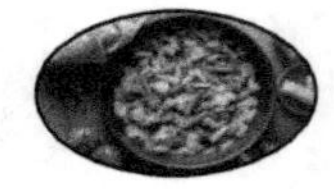

moments spent in the kitchen, savor the flavors that contribute to your well-being, and celebrate the strength that arises from the conscious decision to prioritize health.

This is not merely a conclusion; it is an invitation to a new beginning—a future marked by resilience, vitality, and a commitment to nurturing the body and spirit. May these recipes serve as a constant reminder that, no matter the challenges, you have the power to create a life filled with nourishment, joy, and an abundance of well-deserved victories.

Wishing you a future brimming with health, happiness, and the comforting embrace of anticancer choices. Cheers to a nourished and vibrant life ahead!

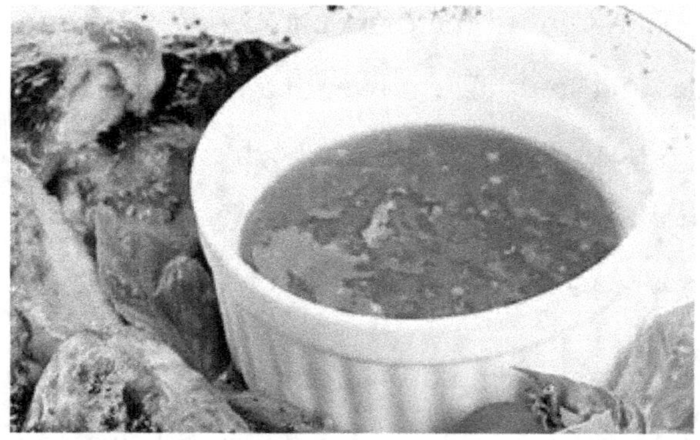

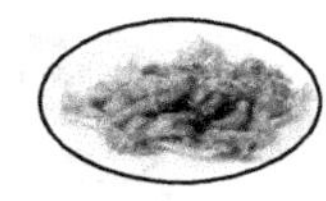 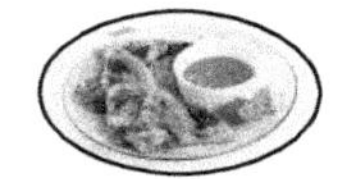 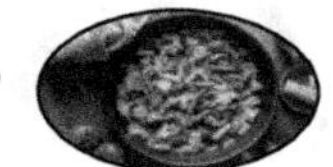

WE KNOW…

THAT'S WHY WE ARE SAYING THANK YOU…

"We know time is the unit of destiny, that's why we are saying thank you."

Dear Valued Customer,

we understand that time is a precious commodity, and we sincerely appreciate you choosing to spend a portion of it with us. Your decision to trust us with your purchase means the world to us, and we want to express our deepest gratitude.

Your support not only fuels our passion for delivering quality products but also contributes to the destiny of our business. Each customer is a vital part of our journey, and we are honored to have you

We strive to provide an exceptional shopping experience, and your satisfaction is our top priority. If you have any feedback or suggestions, we would love to hear from you. Your insights help us improve.

As a small token of our appreciation, we kindly invite you to share your experience by leaving a 5-star review. Your feedback not only boosts our morale but also assists fellow shoppers in making informed decisions.

Once again, thank you for choosing to buy this book. We look forward to serving you again and being a part of your destiny in the world of quality and excellence.

Warm regards,

Dr. Grace Hester

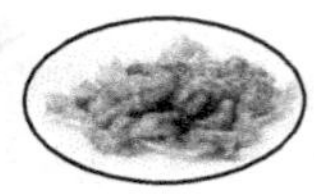 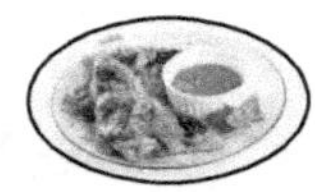 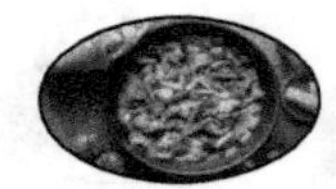

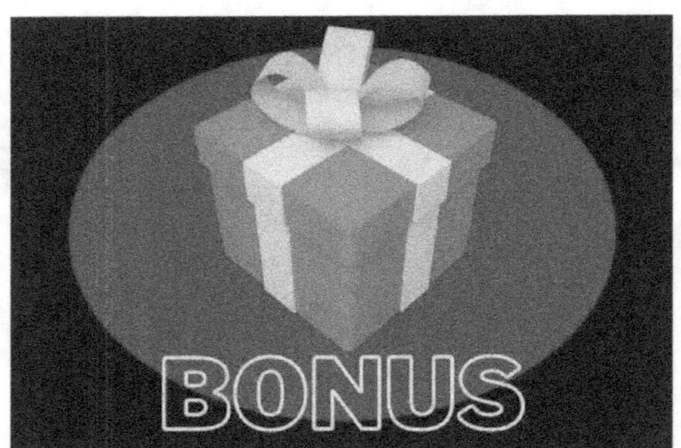

20 DAYS + MEAL PLANNER

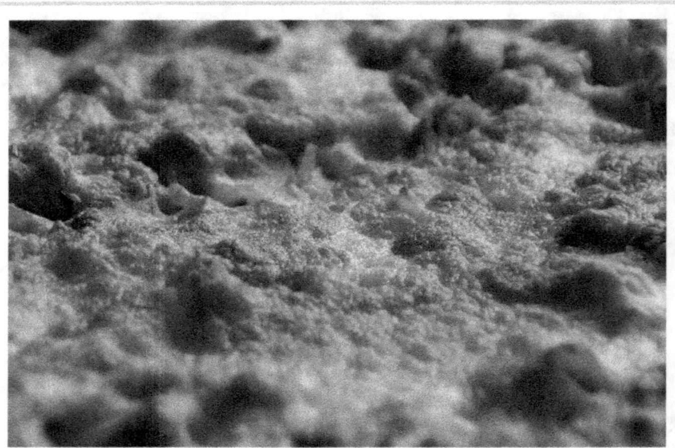

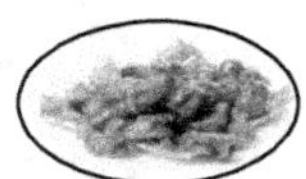
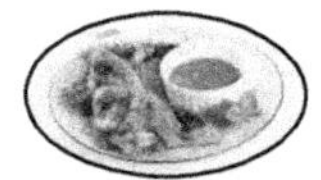
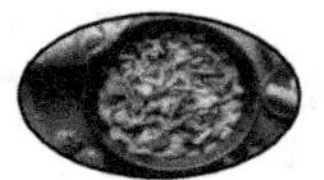

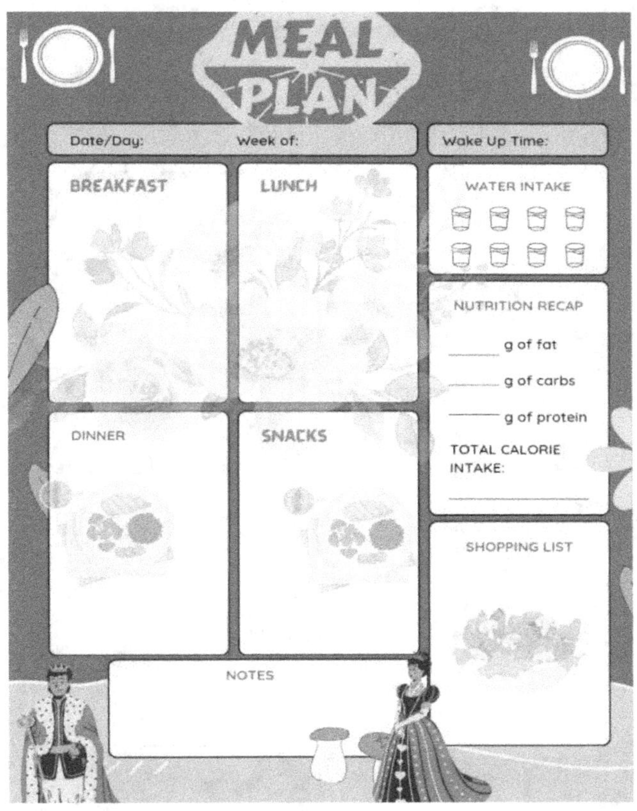
MEAL PLAN
Date/Day:
Week of:
Wake Up Time:
BREAKFAST
LUNCH
WATER INTAKE
NUTRITION RECAP
g of fat
g of carbs
g of protein
TOTAL CALORIE INTAKE:
DINNER
SNACKS
SHOPPING LIST
NOTES

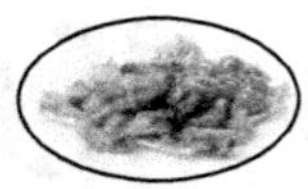 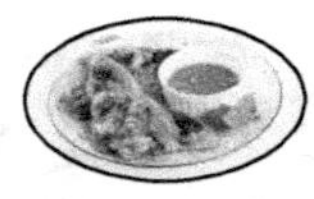 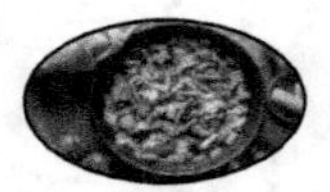

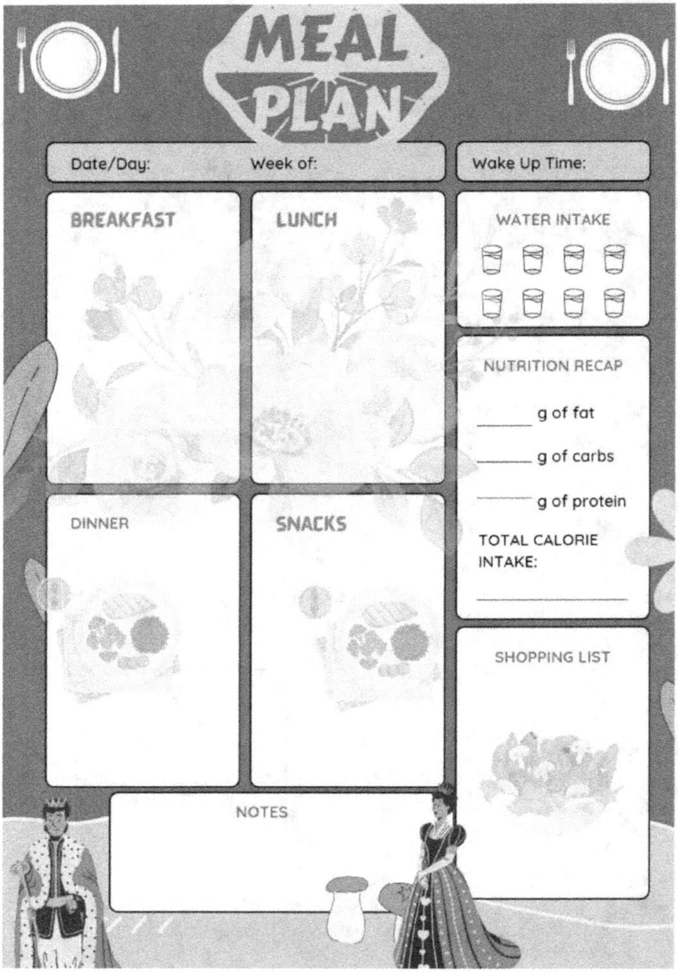

MEAL PLAN

| Date/Day: | Week of: | Wake Up Time: |

BREAKFAST

LUNCH

WATER INTAKE

NUTRITION RECAP

_______ g of fat

_______ g of carbs

_______ g of protein

TOTAL CALORIE INTAKE:

____

DINNER

SNACKS

SHOPPING LIST

NOTES

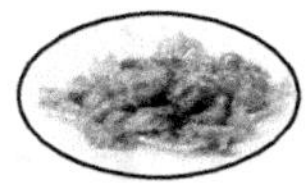 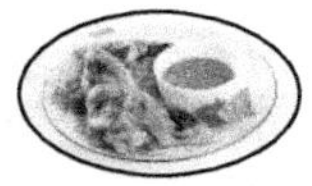 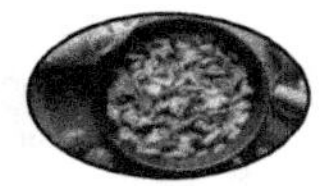

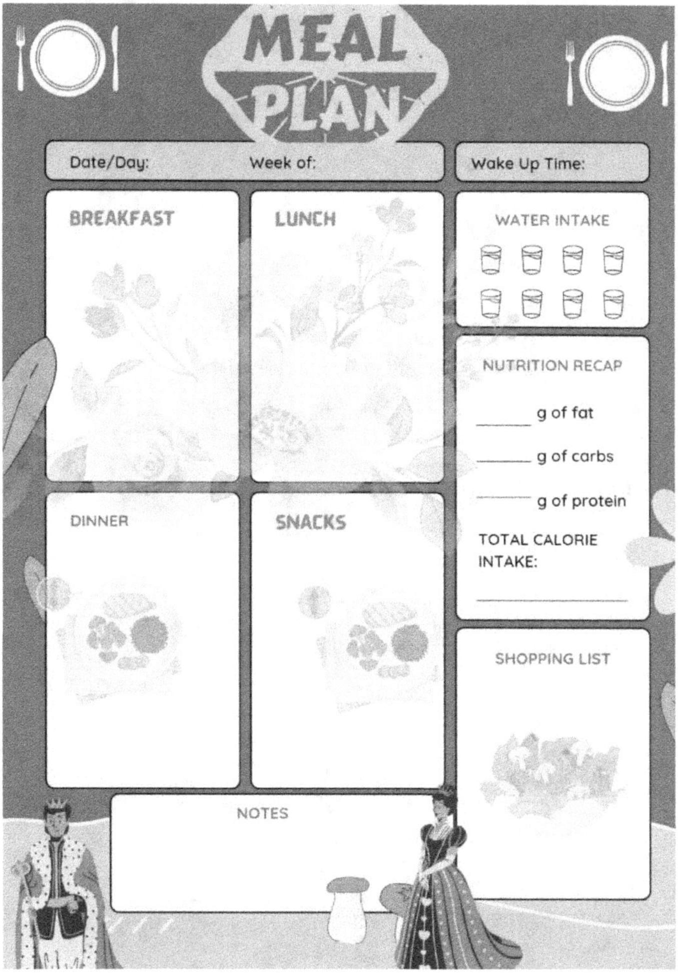

MEAL PLAN

| Date/Day: | Week of: | Wake Up Time: |

BREAKFAST

LUNCH

WATER INTAKE

NUTRITION RECAP

_______ g of fat

_______ g of carbs

_______ g of protein

TOTAL CALORIE INTAKE:

____

DINNER

SNACKS

SHOPPING LIST

NOTES

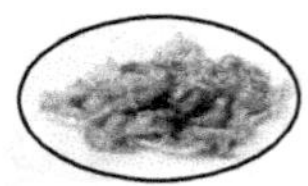 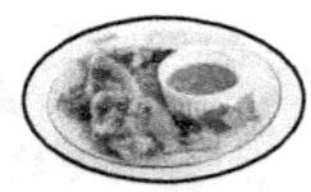 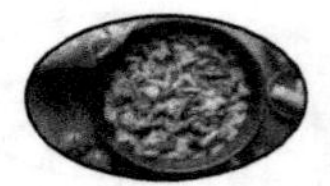

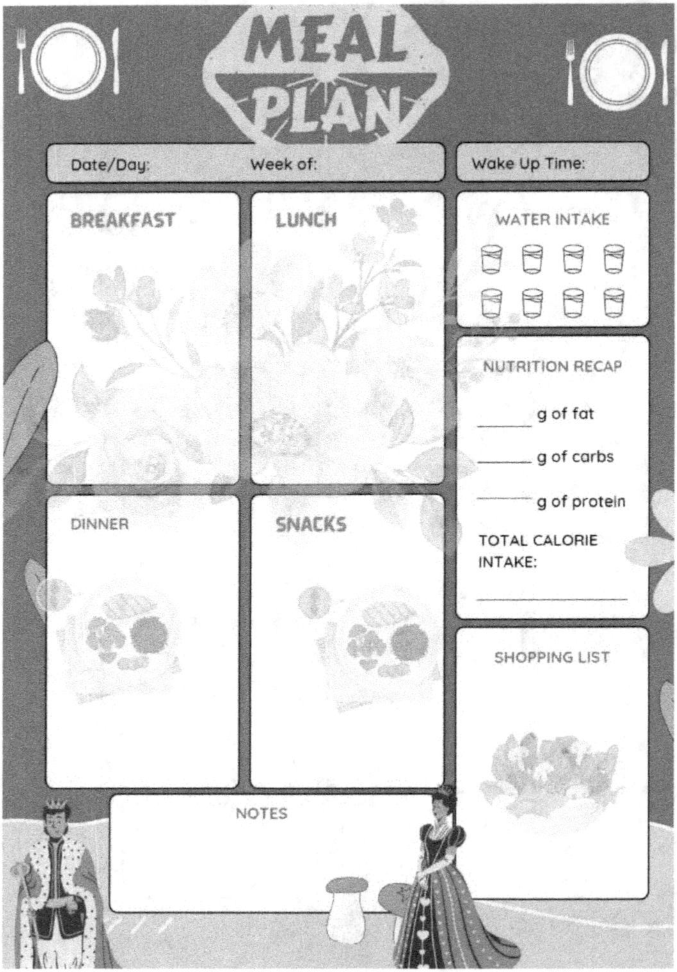

MEAL PLAN

| Date/Day: | Week of: | Wake Up Time: |

BREAKFAST

LUNCH

WATER INTAKE

NUTRITION RECAP

_______ g of fat

_______ g of carbs

_______ g of protein

TOTAL CALORIE INTAKE:

____

DINNER

SNACKS

SHOPPING LIST

NOTES

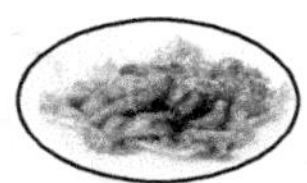 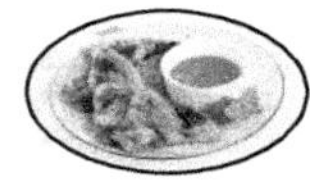 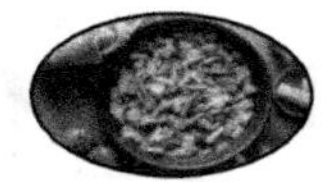

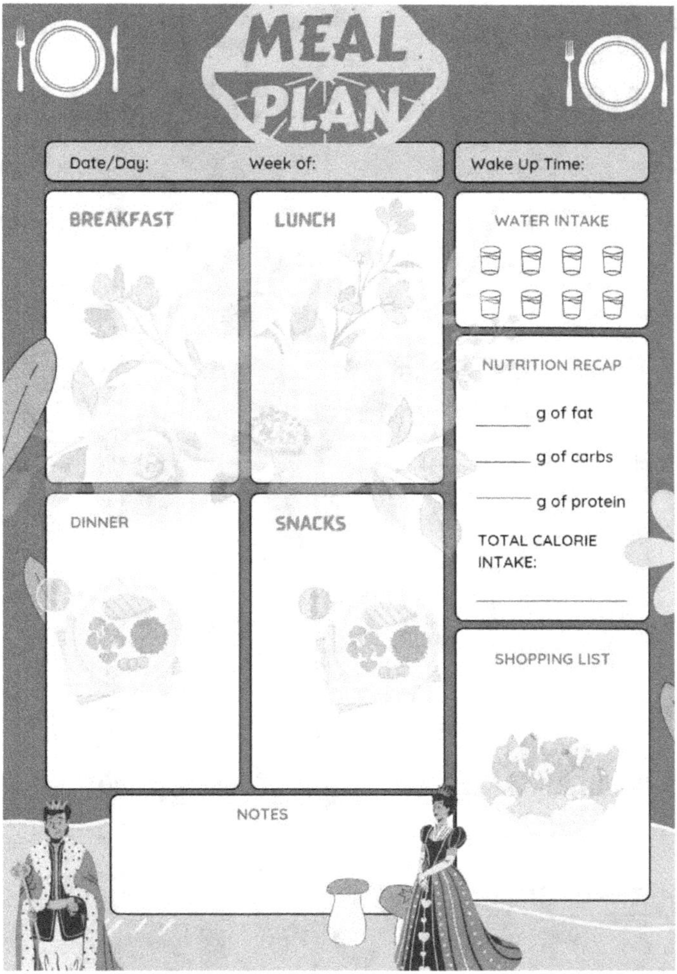

MEAL PLAN

Date/Day:	Week of:	Wake Up Time:

BREAKFAST

LUNCH

WATER INTAKE

NUTRITION RECAP

__________ g of fat

__________ g of carbs

__________ g of protein

TOTAL CALORIE INTAKE:

____

DINNER

SNACKS

SHOPPING LIST

NOTES

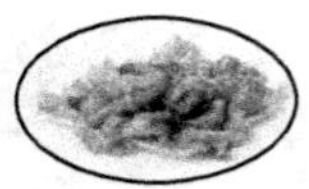 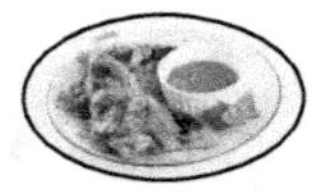 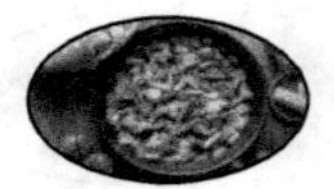

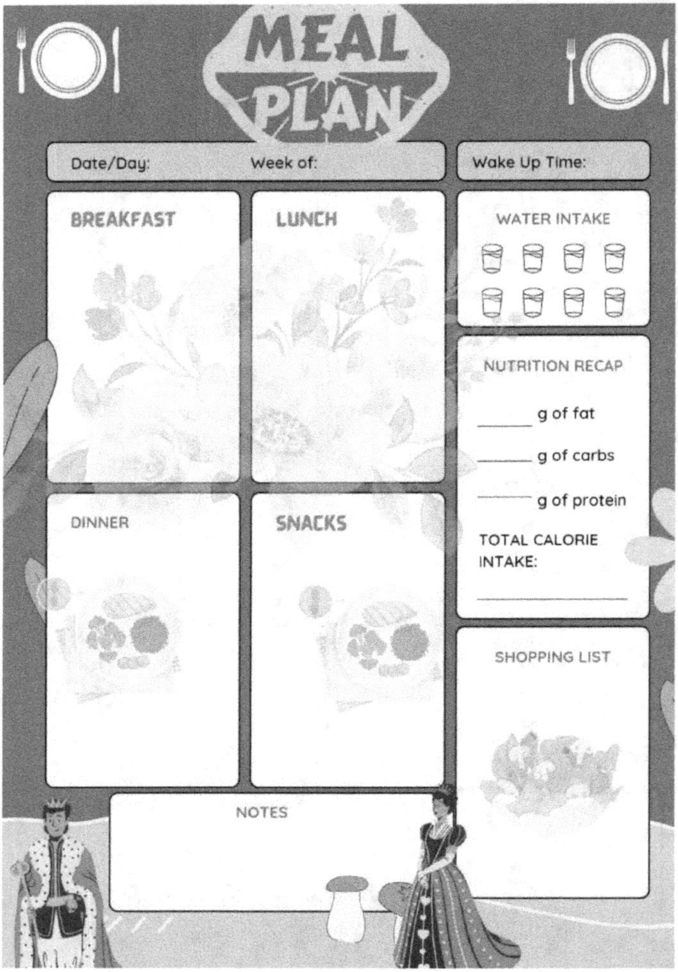

MEAL PLAN

| Date/Day: | Week of: | Wake Up Time: |

BREAKFAST

LUNCH

WATER INTAKE

NUTRITION RECAP

________ g of fat

________ g of carbs

________ g of protein

TOTAL CALORIE INTAKE:

____

DINNER

SNACKS

SHOPPING LIST

NOTES

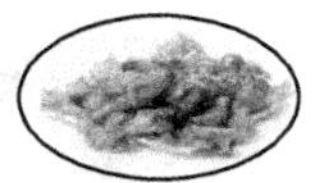 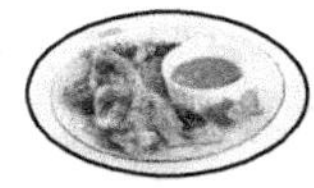 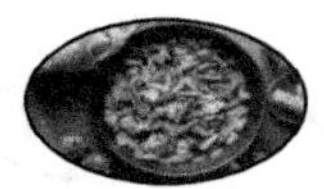

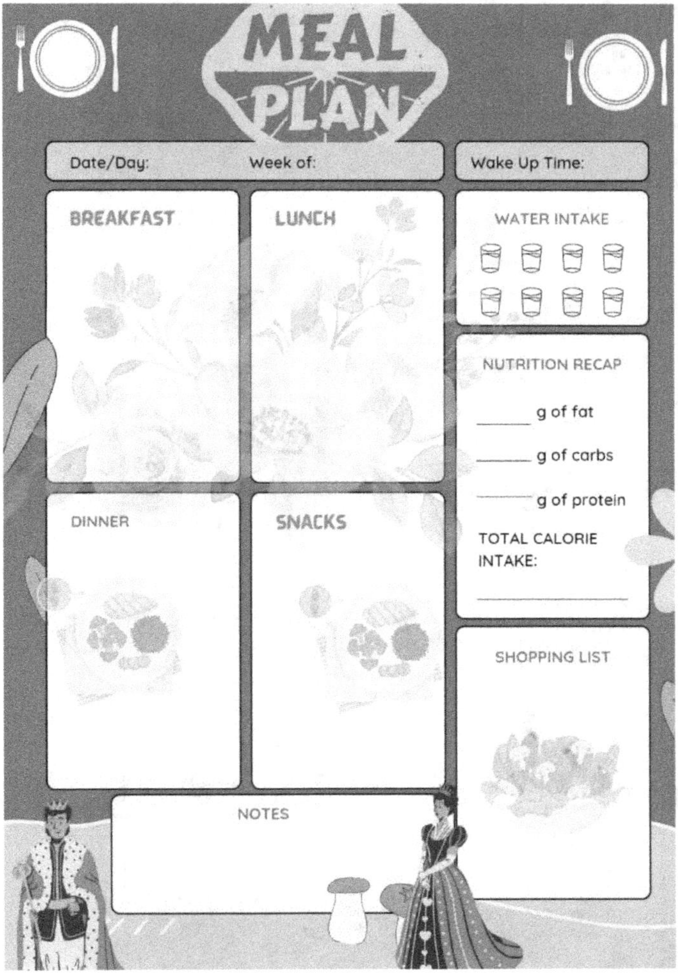

MEAL PLAN

| Date/Day: | Week of: | Wake Up Time: |

BREAKFAST

LUNCH

WATER INTAKE

NUTRITION RECAP

_______ g of fat

_______ g of carbs

_______ g of protein

TOTAL CALORIE INTAKE:

____

DINNER

SNACKS

SHOPPING LIST

NOTES

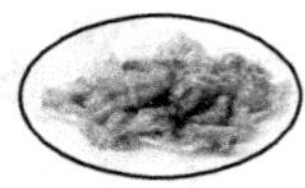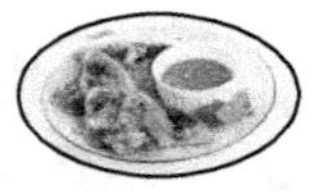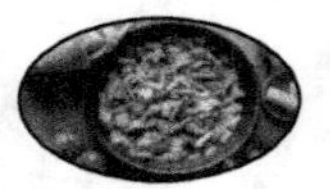

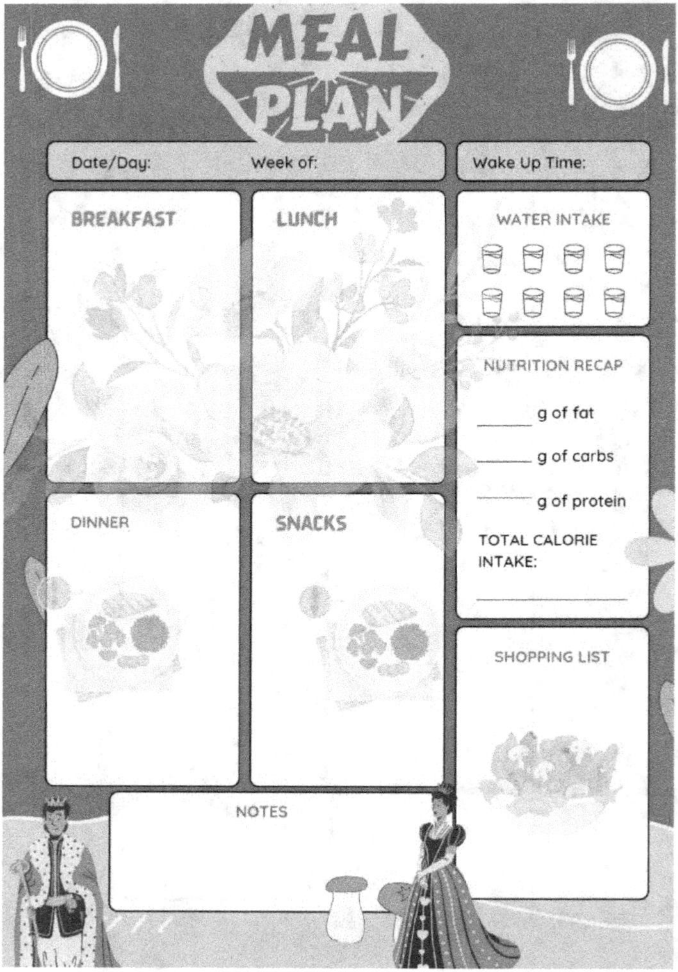

MEAL PLAN

| Date/Day: | Week of: | Wake Up Time: |

BREAKFAST

LUNCH

WATER INTAKE

NUTRITION RECAP

_______ g of fat

_______ g of carbs

_______ g of protein

TOTAL CALORIE INTAKE:

____

DINNER

SNACKS

SHOPPING LIST

NOTES

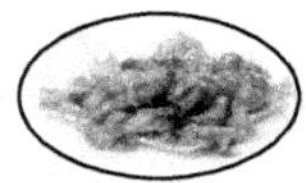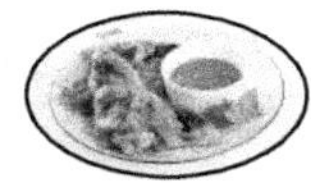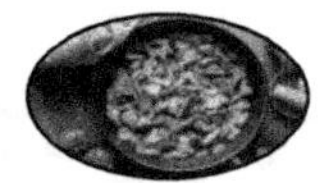

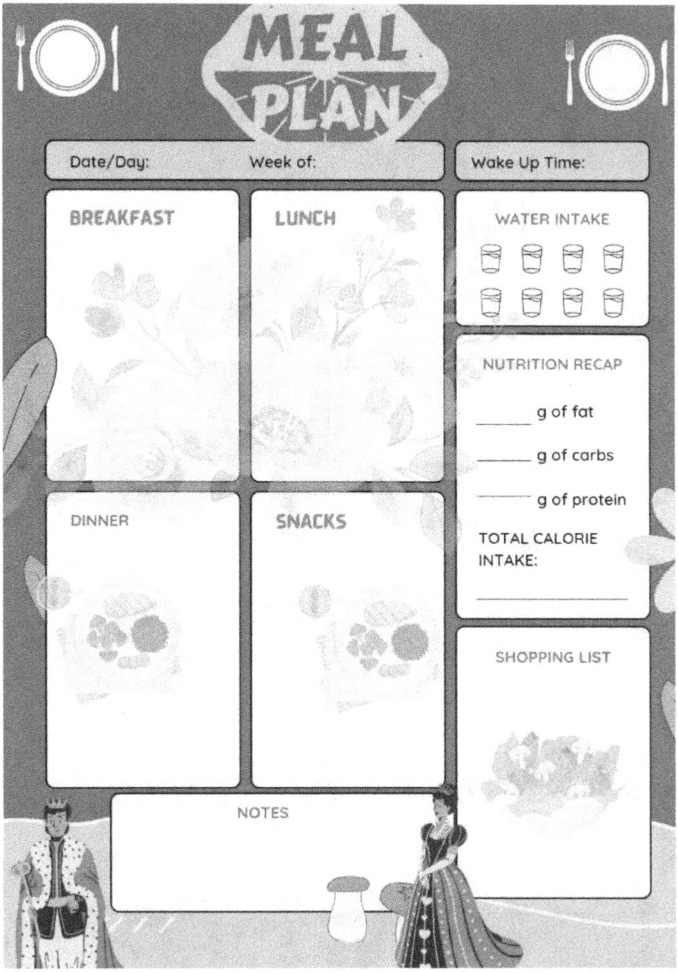

MEAL PLAN

| Date/Day: | Week of: | Wake Up Time: |

BREAKFAST

LUNCH

WATER INTAKE

NUTRITION RECAP

_______ g of fat

_______ g of carbs

_______ g of protein

TOTAL CALORIE INTAKE:

____

DINNER

SNACKS

SHOPPING LIST

NOTES

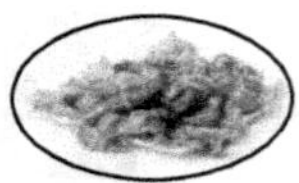 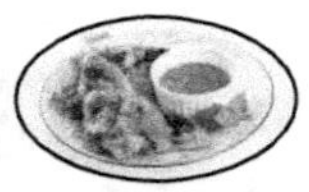 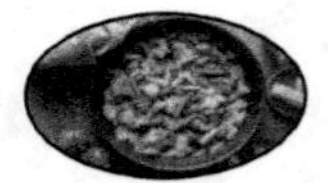

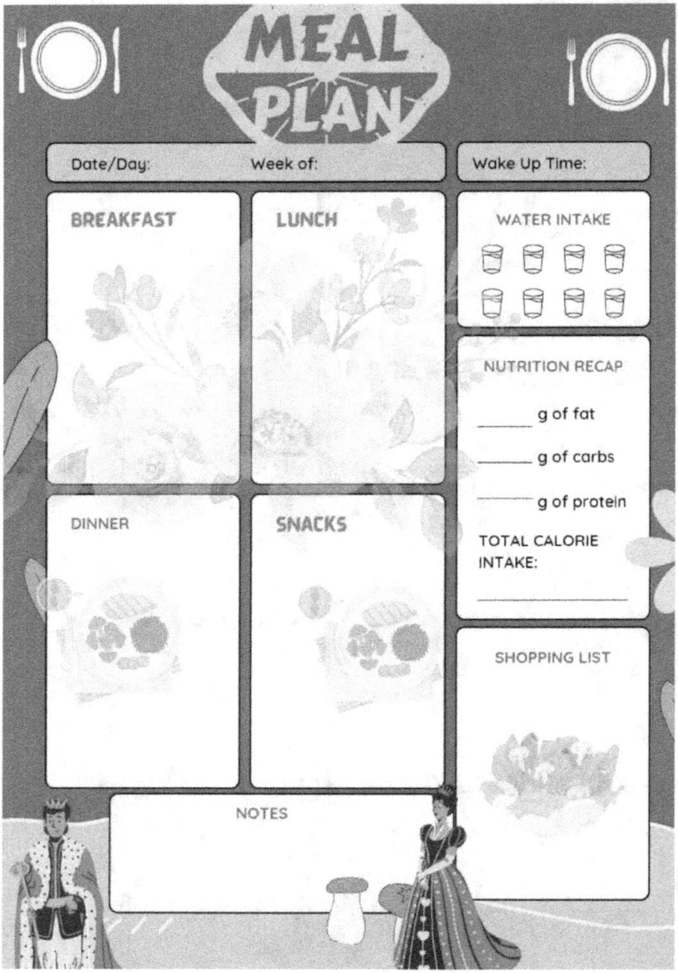

MEAL PLAN

Date/Day:	Week of:	Wake Up Time:

BREAKFAST

LUNCH

WATER INTAKE

NUTRITION RECAP

________ g of fat

________ g of carbs

________ g of protein

TOTAL CALORIE INTAKE:

____

DINNER

SNACKS

SHOPPING LIST

NOTES

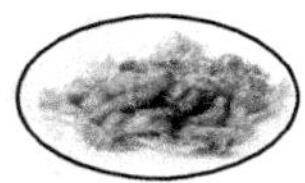 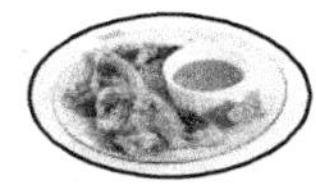 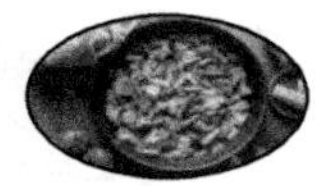

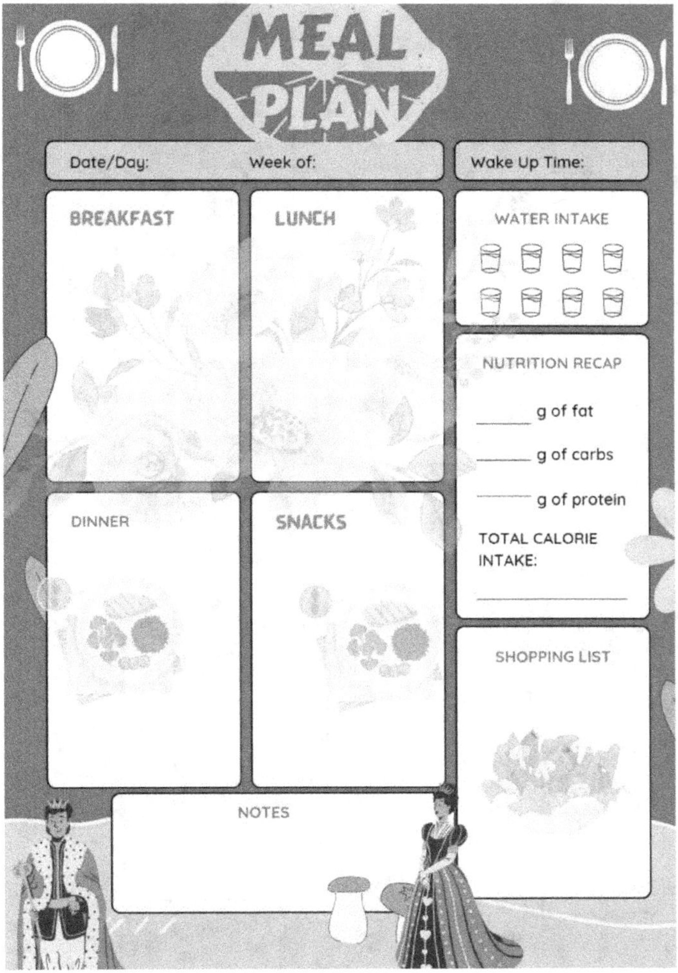

MEAL PLAN

| Date/Day: | Week of: | Wake Up Time: |

BREAKFAST

LUNCH

WATER INTAKE

NUTRITION RECAP

_______ g of fat

_______ g of carbs

_______ g of protein

TOTAL CALORIE INTAKE:

____

DINNER

SNACKS

SHOPPING LIST

NOTES

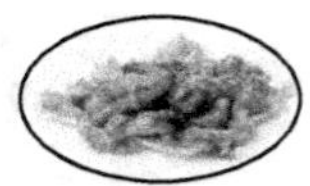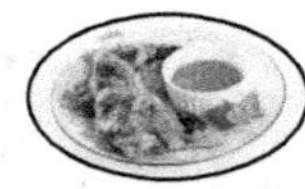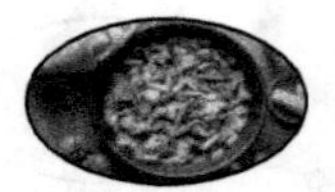

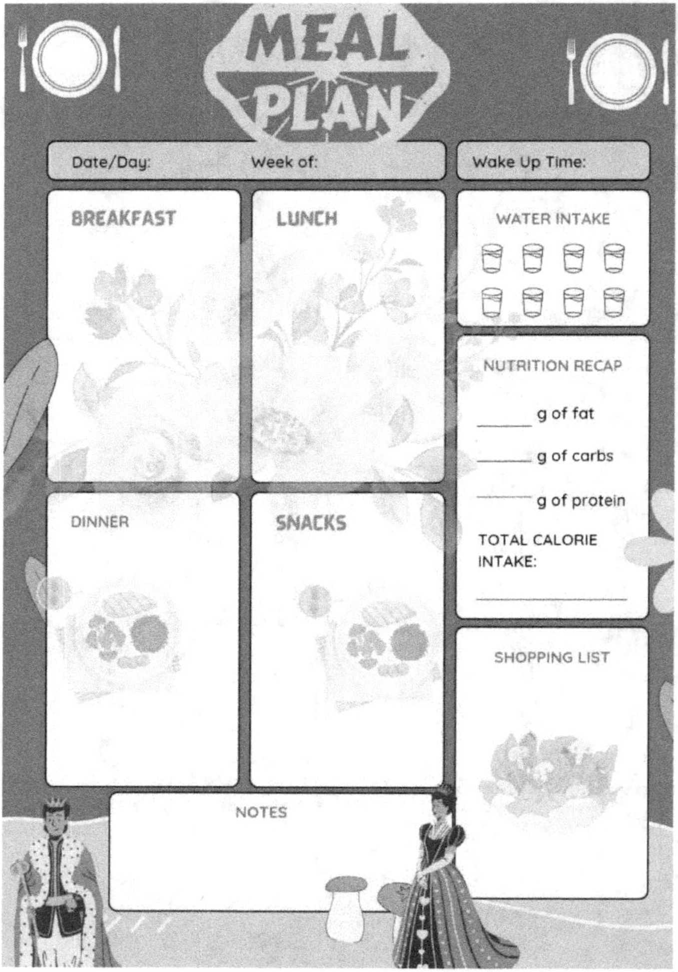

MEAL PLAN

Date/Day:	Week of:	Wake Up Time:

BREAKFAST

LUNCH

WATER INTAKE

NUTRITION RECAP

________ g of fat

________ g of carbs

________ g of protein

TOTAL CALORIE INTAKE:

____

DINNER

SNACKS

SHOPPING LIST

NOTES

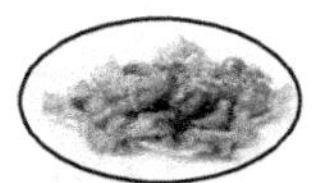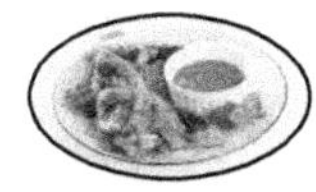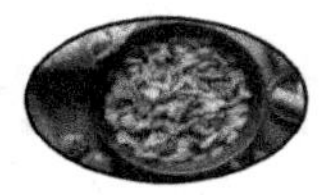

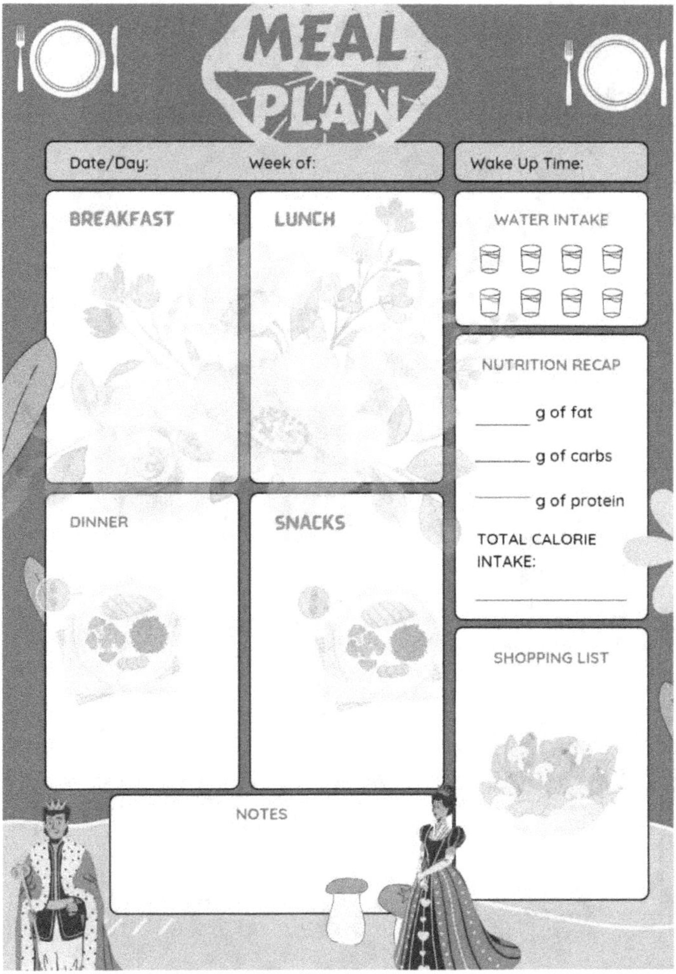

MEAL PLAN

| Date/Day: | Week of: | Wake Up Time: |

BREAKFAST

LUNCH

WATER INTAKE

NUTRITION RECAP

_______ g of fat

_______ g of carbs

_______ g of protein

TOTAL CALORIE
INTAKE:

____

DINNER

SNACKS

SHOPPING LIST

NOTES

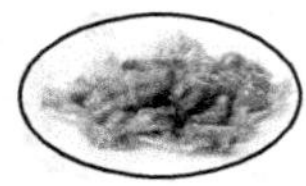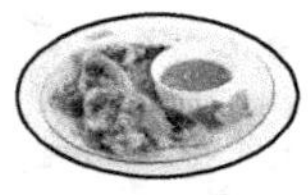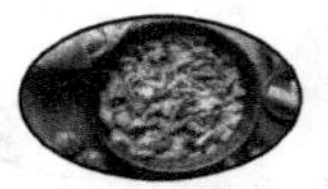

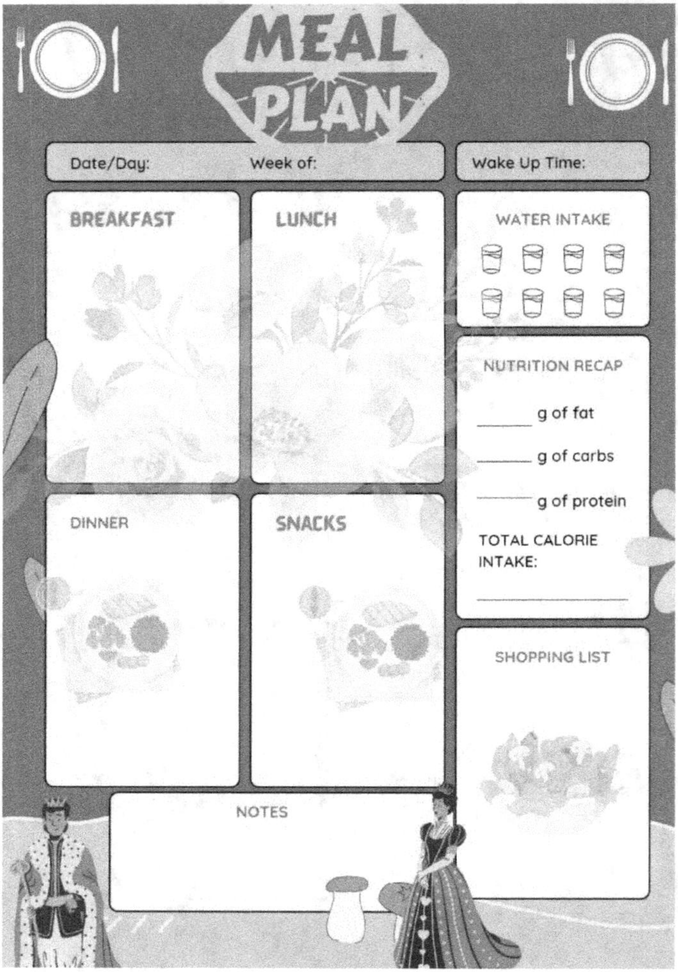

MEAL PLAN

| Date/Day: | Week of: | Wake Up Time: |

BREAKFAST

LUNCH

WATER INTAKE

NUTRITION RECAP

__________ g of fat

__________ g of carbs

__________ g of protein

TOTAL CALORIE INTAKE:

____

DINNER

SNACKS

SHOPPING LIST

NOTES

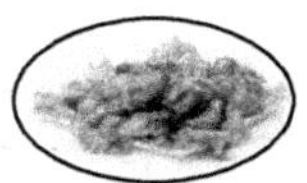 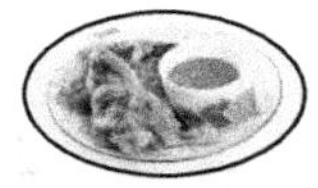 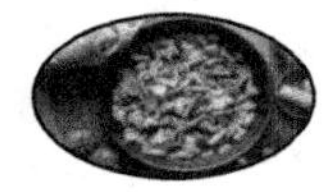

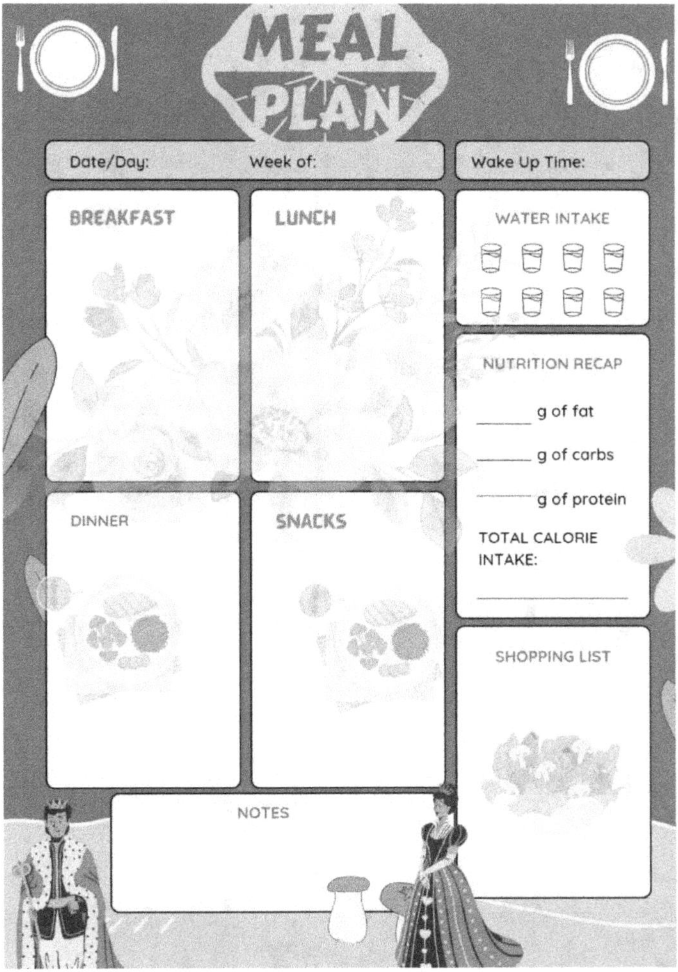

MEAL PLAN

| Date/Day: | Week of: | Wake Up Time: |

BREAKFAST

LUNCH

WATER INTAKE

NUTRITION RECAP

_______ g of fat

_______ g of carbs

_______ g of protein

TOTAL CALORIE INTAKE:

____

DINNER

SNACKS

SHOPPING LIST

NOTES

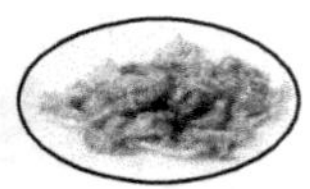 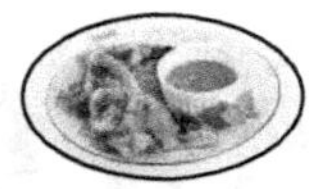 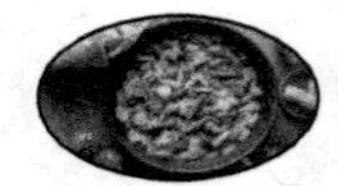

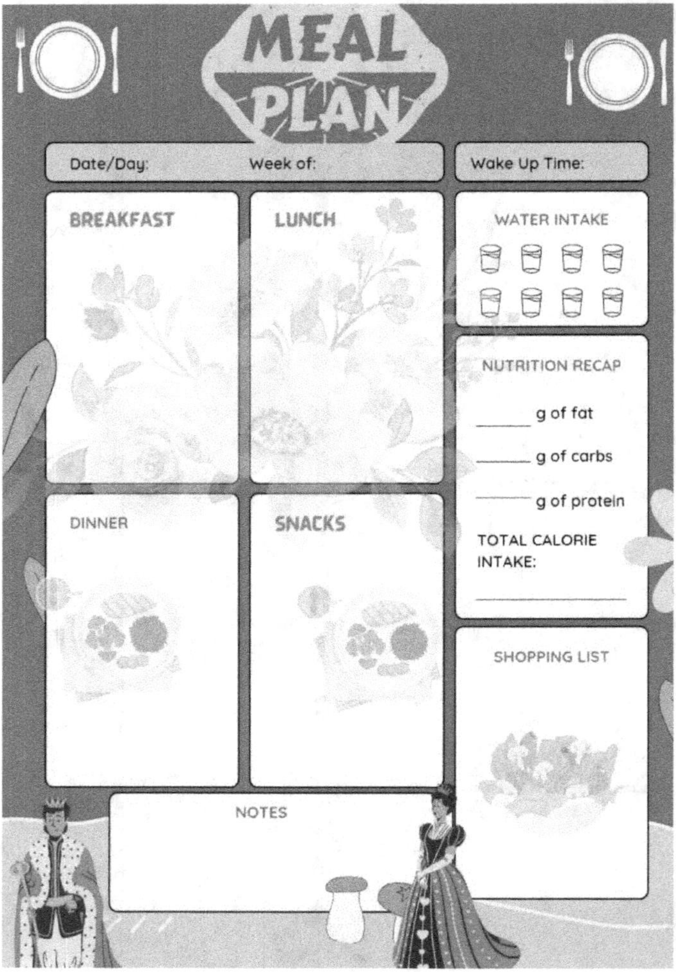

MEAL PLAN

| Date/Day: | Week of: | Wake Up Time: |

BREAKFAST

LUNCH

WATER INTAKE

NUTRITION RECAP

________ g of fat

________ g of carbs

________ g of protein

TOTAL CALORIE INTAKE:

____

DINNER

SNACKS

SHOPPING LIST

NOTES

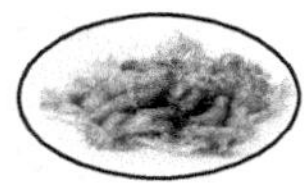 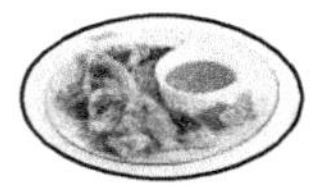 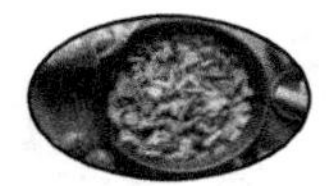

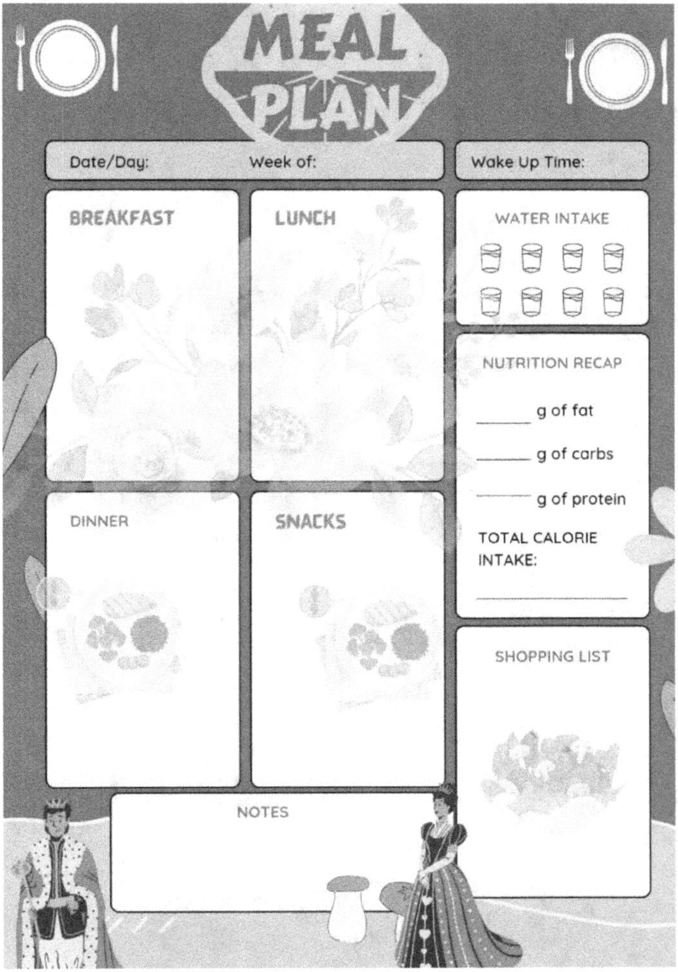

MEAL PLAN

Date/Day: Week of: Wake Up Time:

BREAKFAST

LUNCH

DINNER

SNACKS

WATER INTAKE

NUTRITION RECAP

_________ g of fat

_________ g of carbs

_________ g of protein

TOTAL CALORIE INTAKE:

____

SHOPPING LIST

NOTES

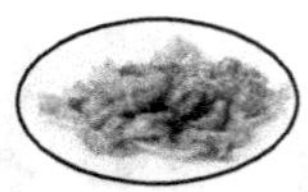 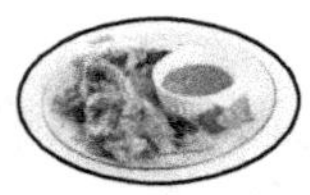 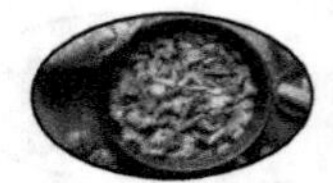

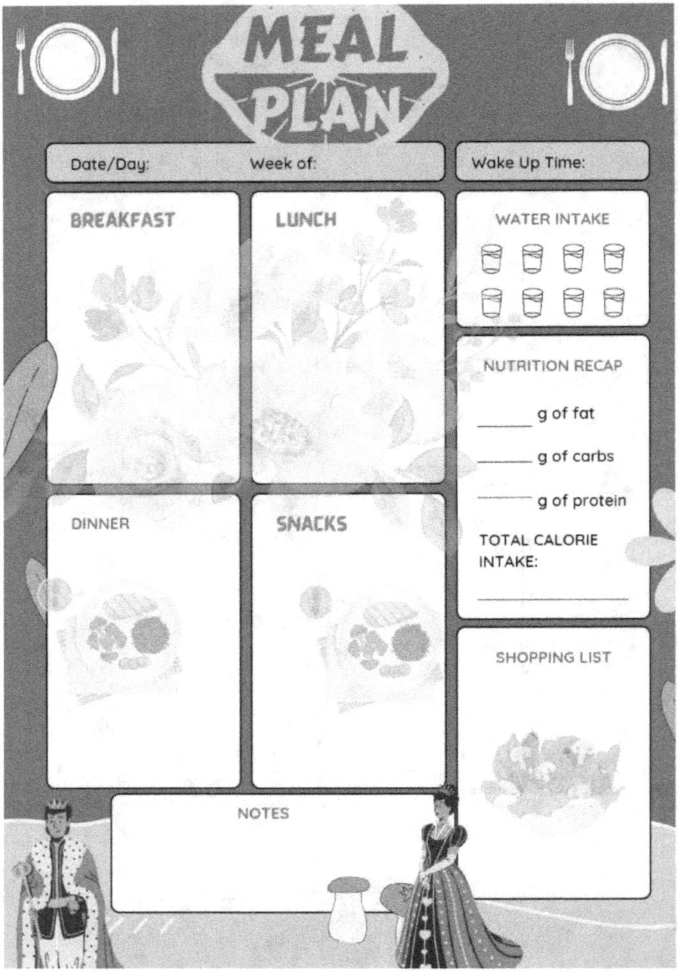

MEAL PLAN

| Date/Day: | Week of: | Wake Up Time: |

BREAKFAST

LUNCH

WATER INTAKE

NUTRITION RECAP

________ g of fat

________ g of carbs

________ g of protein

TOTAL CALORIE INTAKE:

____

DINNER

SNACKS

SHOPPING LIST

NOTES

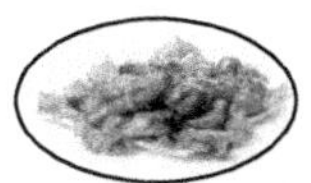 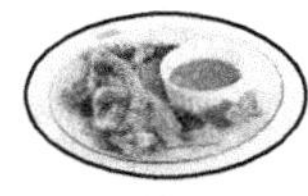 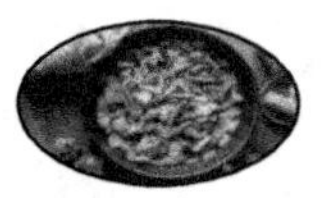

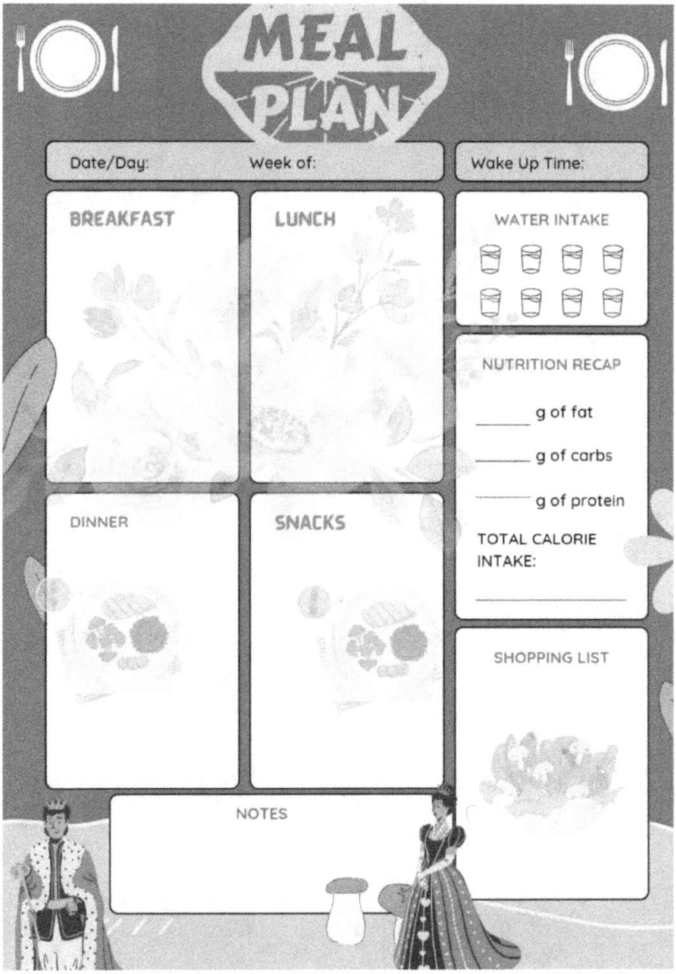

MEAL PLAN

| Date/Day: | Week of: | Wake Up Time: |

BREAKFAST

LUNCH

WATER INTAKE

NUTRITION RECAP

________ g of fat

________ g of carbs

________ g of protein

TOTAL CALORIE INTAKE:

____

DINNER

SNACKS

SHOPPING LIST

NOTES